T0362526

Patent Foramen Ovale

Editor

JONATHAN M. TOBIS

CARDIOLOGY CLINICS

www.cardiology.theclinics.com

November 2024 • Volume 42 • Number 4

ELSEVIER

1600 John F. Kennedy Boulevard • Suite 1800 • Philadelphia, Pennsylvania, 19103-2899

http://www.theclinics.com

CARDIOLOGY CLINICS Volume 42, Number 4
November 2024 ISSN 0733-8651, ISBN-13: 978-0-443-12969-8

Editor: Joanna Gascoine
Developmental Editor: Malvika Shah

Cardiology Clinics (ISSN 0733-8651) is published quarterly by Elsevier Inc., 360 Park Avenue South, New York, NY 10010-1710. Months of issue are February, May, August, and November. Business and Editorial Offices: 1600 John F. Kennedy Blvd., Ste. 1800, Philadelphia, PA 19103-2899. Customer Service Office: 3251 Riverport Lane, Maryland Heights, MO 63043. Periodicals post-age paid at New York, NY and additional mailing offices. Subscription prices are $396.00 per year for US individuals, $100.00 per year for US students and residents, $472.00 per year for Canadian individuals, $495.00 per year for international individuals, $100.00 per year for Canadian students/residents and $220.00 per year for international students/residents. For institutional access pricing please contact Customer Service via the contact information below. To receive student/resident rate, orders must be accompanied by name of affiliated institution, data of term, and the *signature* of program/residency coordinator on institution letterhead. Orders will be billed at individual rate until proof of status is received. Foreign air speed delivery is included in all *Clinics* subscription prices. All prices are subject to change without notice. Orders, claims, and journal inquiries: Please visit our Support Hub page https://service.elsevier.com for assistance.

Reprints. For copies of 100 or more, of articles in this publication, please contact the Commercial Reprints Department, Elsevier Inc., 360 Park Avenue South, New York, NY 10010-1710. Tel.: 212-633-3874; Fax: 212-633-3820; E-mail: reprints@elsevier.com.

Cardiology Clinics is also published in Spanish by McGraw-Hill Interamericana Editores S. A., P.O. Box 5-237, 06500, Mexico D. F., Mexico; in Portuguese by Reichmann and Alfonso Editores Rio de Janeiro, Brazil; and in Greek by Dimitrios P. Lagos, 8 Pondon Street, GR115-28 Ilissia, Greece.

Cardiology Clinics is covered in *MEDLINE/PubMed (Index Medicus), Excerpta Medica, The Cumulative Index to Nursing and Allied Health Literature* (CINAHL).

Contributors

ADEBA MOHAMMAD, DO, MS
Resident Physician, Cardiology Department, Loma Linda University Health, Loma Linda, California, USA

SANAULLAH MOJADDEDI, MD
University of Central Florida College of Medicine, Graduate Medical Education, Orlando, Florida, USA; Resident, Internal Medicine Residency Program, HCA Florida North Florida Hospital, Gainesville, Florida, USA

MOHAMMAD K. MOJADIDI, MD, FACP, FACC
Assistant Professor, Division of Cardiology, Department of Medicine, Virginia Commonwealth University (VCU Health), Richmond, Virginia, USA

SANJANA NAGRAJ, MBBS
Fellow, Division of Cardiology, Montefiore Medical Center, Albert Einstein College of Medicine, Bronx, New York, USA

ASHLEY NGUYEN, DO
Department of Medicine, Cleveland Clinic Florida, Weston, Florida, USA

ELAINE NGUYEN, MD
Division of Pulmonary and Critical Care Medicine, Department of Medicine, Riverside University Health System, Moreno Valley, California, USA

LEONIDAS PALAIODIMOS, MD, MS, FACP
Department of Medicine, New York City Health + Hospitals/Jacobi, Associate Professor, Division of Hospital Medicine Albert Einstein College of Medicine, Bronx, New York, USA

RUSHI V. PARIKH, MD
Associate Professor, Department of Medicine, Division of Cardiology, University of California Los Angeles, Los Angeles, California, USA

KERSTIN PIAYDA, MD, MSc
Cardiovascular Center Frankfurt, Frankfurt, Germany; Attending cardiologist, Department of Cardiology and Vascular Medicine, University Hospital Gießen and Marburg, Gießen, Germany

DEEPAK RAVI, MD
Clinical Fellow, Department of Medicine, Division of Cardiology, University of California Los Angeles, Los Angeles, California, USA

BARBARA T. ROBBINS, FNP-BC
Nurse Practitioner, Department of Medicine, Division of Interventional Cardiology, Columbia University Medical Center, New York, New York, USA

JEFFREY L. SAVER, MD
Professor and Carol and James Collins Endowed Chair in Neurology, Department of Neurology and Comprehensive Stroke Center, David Geffen School of Medicine, University of California, Los Angeles, Los Angeles, California, USA

ALOK SHARMA, MD
Interventional and Structural Cardiologist, Minneapolis Veterans Affairs Medical Center, Minneapolis, Minnesota, USA

HORST SIEVERT, MD
Director, Cardiovascular Center Frankfurt, Associate Professor of Internal Medicine/Cardiology, University of Frankfurt, Frankfurt, Germany

ROBERT J. SOMMER, MD
Associate Professor, Department of Medicine, Division of Interventional Cardiology, Columbia University Medical Center, New York, New York, USA

JONATHAN M. TOBIS, MD
Professor of Medicine/Cardiology, Department of Medicine, Division of Cardiology, David Geffen School of Medicine at UCLA, University of California Los Angeles, Ronald Reagan UCLA Medical Center, Los Angeles, California, USA

HUUTAM TRUONG, MD, FSCAI
Cardiologist, VA Loma Linda Healthcare System, Loma Linda, California, USA

VERENA VEULEMANS, MD
Cardiologist, Department of Cardiology, Pneumology and Vascular Medicine, University Hospital Düsseldorf, Düsseldorf, Germany

BRIAN WEST, MD
Cardiologist, Sharp Rees-Stealy Medical Group, San Diego, California, USA

MUHAMMAD O. ZAMAN, MD
Department of Cardiovascular Medicine, University of Louisville, University of Louisville Heart Hospital, Louisville, Kentucky, USA

Contents

Video content accompanies this article at http://www.cardiology.theclinics.com.

When it comes to procedural guidance during PFO closure, various modalities exist, each with its own advantages and disadvantages. Guidance by transesophageal echocardiography (in combination with fluoroscopy) offers high-resolution 2D/3D imaging, however, it requires the presence of a peri-interventional imager and conscious sedation (or endotracheal intubation). Intracardiac echocardiography and fluoroscopy guidance can be performed by a single operator and omits the need for conscious sedation (or endotracheal intubation).

 Video content accompanies this article at http://www.cardiology.theclinics.com.

The patent foramen ovale (PFO) jeopardizes health and its problems may be major. A nineteenth century case report was the first description of a PFO as cause of death. To the present day, the PFO does not get the deserved attention. A PFO is found in roughly 25% of people, its particularly dangerous forms in about 5%. Those have a high enough risk for harm by the PFO to justify screening for it for closure, even as primary prevention. After all, closing a PFO is as simple as fixing a tooth and can be considered a mechanical vaccination.

Patent foramen ovale (PFO) may be an underlying factor in the pathogenesis of migraine, vasospastic angina, and Takotsubo cardiomyopathy. This article reviews the role that PFO may play in each of these clinical entities and discusses potential interventions. It also proposes a novel clinical syndrome wherein PFO may be the unifying link among migraine, coronary vasospasm, and Takotsubo cardiomyopathy in predisposed individuals.

CARDIOLOGY CLINICS

SERIES OF RELATED INTEREST

Heart Failure Clinics
Available at: https://www.heartfailure.theclinics.com/
Cardiac Electrophysiology Clinics
Available at: https://www.cardiacep.theclinics.com/
Interventional Cardiology Clinics
Available at: https://www.interventional.theclinics.com/

Dedication

This issue on patent foramen ovale (PFO) is dedicated to my oncologist, Alexandra Drakaki, MD, and the researchers who developed immunotherapy. Without their support, I would not have been alive to help write and edit this compendium on PFO. I had a nephrectomy for renal cell carcinoma in April 2023 and began immunotherapy for metastatic disease in November 2023. I appreciate the opportunity I have been given to describe the research in this field over the past 25 years.

Jonathan M. Tobis, MD
David Geffen School of Medicine at UCLA
Los Angeles, CA, USA

E-mail address:
jtobis@mednet.ucla.edu

Cardiol Clin 42 (2024) ix
https://doi.org/10.1016/j.ccl.2024.02.022

Preface
The Current State of Science Surrounding Patent Foramen Ovale

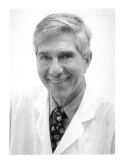

Jonathan M. Tobis, MD
Editor

The exploration of patent foramen ovale (PFO) as a pathway for multiple disease states has been one of the more fascinating advances in cardiology over the last 25 years. This compendium of articles describe some of the major issues and clinical states surrounding the study of PFOs. The authors who wrote these articles are some of the leading people in this field. They deserve much credit for helping us understand the sometimes subtle mechanisms associated with PFO. It is our hope that this collection of articles will help educate neurologists and cardiologists who deal with PFO-associated clinical situations, such as stroke of unknown cause, migraine with aura, decompression illness, altitude sickness, and hypoxemia out of proportion to the degree of pulmonary disease. We hope these articles provide practical information that will be useful to clinicians and help them understand some of the nuances of making the diagnosis and options for treatment of PFO-related problems.

DISCLOSURES

Dr J.M. Tobis is a consultant and proctor for WL Gore, Inc.

Jonathan M. Tobis, MD
David Geffen School of Medicine at UCLA
Los Angeles, CA, USA

E-mail address:
jtobis@mednet.ucla.edu

Cardiol Clin 42 (2024) xi
https://doi.org/10.1016/j.ccl.2024.01.002
0733-8651/24/© 2024 Published by Elsevier Inc.

Some Practical Points About Patent Foramen Ovale Conditions that May Not Be Covered in the Rest of the Book

Jonathan M. Tobis, MD

KEYWORDS

• Patent foramen ovale • Stroke • Migraine • Altitude sickness

KEY POINTS

• The gold standard for diagnosing a patent foramen ovale (PFO) should be a right heart catheterization with proof that a guidewire or catheter has traversed the atrial septum.
• The PFO-Associated Stroke Causal Likelihood (PASCAL) classification system should be used by neurologists to determine whether the PFO is likely to be causally related to the stroke or an "innocent association."
• "PFO Associated Stroke" is now considered a separate entity as a cause of stroke, which should facilitate the workup and treatment option for this condition.

INTRODUCTION

The exploration of patent foramen ovale (PFO) as a pathway for multiple disease states has been one of the more fascinating advances in cardiology over the last 25 years. This compendium of articles will describe some of the major clinical conditions and issues surrounding the study of PFO. The authors who wrote these chapters are some of the leading experts in this field. They deserve much credit for helping us understand the sometimes subtle mechanisms associated with PFO. It is our hope that this collection of articles will help educate neurologists and cardiologists who deal with PFO-associated clinical states such as stroke of otherwise unknown etiology, migraine with aura, decompression illness, altitude sickness, and hypoxemia out of proportion to underlying pulmonary disease. We hope that these chapters provide useful information for clinicians, helping them understand some of the nuances of PFO diagnosis, and treatment options for PFO-related conditions.

As with all doctors, I first learned about PFO in medical school embryology and anatomy and then revisited it as a cardiology fellow to understand fetal physiology. But I only learned that a PFO could cause pathologic states when I heard a lecture by Jim Locke, from Boston Children's Hospital, at the American College of Cardiology meeting around 1998. I was fascinated that a common cardiac structure was only now being associated with stroke in young otherwise healthy individuals. I was hooked by Jim's magnetic delivery and wanted to get involved in this field to understand it better. In 2001, I was visited by Rudy Davis at University of California, Los Angeles (UCLA), who was working on the development of the CardioSeal device by NMT Medical (Boston, MA). The technology advanced significantly with the Amplatzer PFO occluder (Abbott; Chicago, IL) developed by Kurt Amplatz. Subsequent technological improvements were made by W.L. Gore & Associates (Newark, DE) with the Helex and then the Cardioform devices. Instead of being

David Geffen School of Medicine at UCLA, Los Angeles, CA, USA
E-mail address: jtobis@mednet.ucla.edu

Cardiol Clin 42 (2024) 455–461
https://doi.org/10.1016/j.ccl.2024.01.003
0733-8651/24/

a rare entity, I have seen over 1200 patients with PFO-associated conditions that are described in this book. The fact that patients like these were not identified prior to the 1990s provides a lesson in the history of medical science. It was only with new diagnostic tools such as modern echocardiography, equipped with harmonic imaging and transesophageal echo with injection of contrast that these right-to-left shunts were more readily identified in vivo.

Cryptogenic Stroke Versus Patent Foramen Ovale-associated Stroke: What Is in a Name?

One of the benefits of the isolation imposed by the coronavirus-19 pandemic was that it permitted the virtual convening of a working group of cardiologists and neurologists who were involved in PFO research. The purpose of this group was to recognize the advances that have been made over the last 20 years in identifying the causality of PFO related to many strokes of otherwise unknown etiology. Instead of calling these "cryptogenic strokes," the group felt confident that there were enough data to assign this category of stroke as "PFO associated stroke."[1] The nomenclature change is important because it recognizes that a PFO can be pathologically involved as a pathway for stroke, rather than an uncertain consideration when all other causes are ruled out. In addition, naming PFO as a subcategory of stroke has helped to formalize the workup and evaluation of these patients. At UCLA, the stroke neurologists are usually the physicians who first see these patients and evaluate them with a transcranial Doppler (TCD), because this is the most sensitive screening method to identify right-to-left shunt. If that is positive, they obtain a transesophageal echocardiogram (TEE) to identify if there are high-risk aspects of the PFO such as an atrial septal aneurysm. The TCD also quantitates the shunt severity. This information, together with the clinical evaluation, has led to the PASCAL classification which helps to stratify the likelihood that the stroke was due to the PFO pathway.[2]

Pearls and Pitfalls: Some Practical Points About Patent Foramen Ovale

Although autopsy studies demonstrate a probe patent or larger PFO in 35% of cases, I define a clinically significant right-to-left shunt as a grade 3 or larger shunt on a TCD study. This degree of shunting on TCD corresponds to a moderate size ($\geq$6 mm) PFO by balloon sizing during cardiac catheterization. In our control population of 200 unselected people referred to the cardiac catheterization laboratory (excluding known congenital heart disease or transplant patients), we found this degree of shunting in 20% of subjects. PFO is thus the most common form of congenital heart lesion. There are data to suggest that PFO is hereditary, although it is not a direct autosomal dominant inheritance (Tobis, Gevorgian, and West, unpublished data from UCLA). In a study of 154 patients from 50 families, the incidence of PFO was 63% among first-degree relatives.

A foramen ovale is essential for fetal survival because the amount of oxygen delivered through the placenta is only 67% saturated. If this degree of desaturated blood, coming from the placental veins to the inferior vena cava, was to be pumped through the nonfunctioning fetal lungs, the blood would lose more oxygen and there would be insufficient oxygen delivery for fetal survival. The PFO permits placental blood to pass directly across the atrial septum and enter the arterial circulation. This mechanism is so important that it is preserved throughout evolution. All mammals must have a PFO.

Echocardiographic Bubble Studies and the Best Way to Diagnose a Patent Foramen Ovale

One consideration that is frustrating about this field is the disconnect between echocardiographic assessment of right-to-left shunts and what is observed in the catheterization laboratory. The echocardiography literature is replete with studies comparing transthoracic echocardiography (TTE) with TEE or even TCD. The literature considers TEE to be the gold standard. But the TTE and TEE assessment of the severity of the shunt or the size of the PFO is often misleading when compared to balloon sizing measurements made in the catheterization laboratory.[3–8] The echo report may say that the PFO size is small, with the implication that the PFO would be too small to permit a thrombus to pass through and cause the patient's stroke. But during cardiac catheterization, the PFO may be an average size (7 mm) or larger. In support of this observation, a pooled analysis of 2 clinical trials of "high-risk" PFO closure for stroke (ie, studies that only closed PFOs of stroke patients with a large shunt or atrial septal aneurysm) found that although an atrial septal aneurysm was a significant predictor of recurrent stroke, a large shunt by echocardiography was not.[9] I believe that these studies are likely incorrectly categorizing some patients' PFOs as "small" based on echocardiography data alone.

A similar mistake occurs for the echocardiographic assessment of the timing of agitated saline bubbles arriving to the left atrium. Contrary to most echocardiographic literature statements, delayed arrival does not mean that there is a pulmonary arterial-venous malformation (AVM) shunt. It may take time for the bubbles to fill the superior aspect of the right atrium near the fossa ovalis and the PFO does not open up in every cardiac cycle. In our experience with over 2000 TCD examinations, a PFO was present 99% of the time in cases where there was a significant shunt (TCD $\geq$ grade 3) versus 1% for a pulmonary AVM. If a patient has hereditary hemorrhagic telangiectasia, then the incidence of pulmonary AVM is 30%, but these cases are infrequent.[10] I would caution physicians who are interested in this field to be skeptical of the echocardiographic data that does not compare the frequency of finding a PFO with evidence based on a right heart catheterization (ie, ability to pass a guidewire across the atrial septum), which should be the correct in vivo gold standard for PFO diagnosis. I hope that the echocardiographic societies will reassess their guideline statements, as TEE (the current accepted gold standard by echocardiographic societies) can miss or misdiagnose a PFO in 10% of cases.[7]

Patent Foramen Ovale-Associated Stroke

Other chapters will focus on the randomized clinical trials which demonstrated that PFO closure is preferable to medical therapy for prevention of recurrent strokes. I will limit my comments to some curious incidental observations about PFO-associated stroke. Based on the number of ischemic strokes of unknown origin and the frequency of PFO in the population, it is estimated that the risk of a PFO-associated stroke is approximately 1 in 1000 patients with a PFO per year. In patients who present with PFO-associated stroke, the recurrence rate increases 10-fold to 1% per year on medical therapy. The longest clinical trials followed patients for 10 years and the repeat incidence of stroke was 10% in the medically treated arm.[11] It is likely that these patients self-select for those who have an increased likelihood of developing venous thrombosis, presumably from varicose veins or hemorrhoids.

Some of the patients have a predisposition to form a venous thrombus, usually from a congenital abnormality in the clotting cascade. But the predominant form of thrombophilia is acquired, with the use of estrogen-containing compounds either for birth control or hormone replacement therapy.[12] In one of our series, 50% of women who had a PFO-associated stroke were on estrogen therapy at the time of their event.[13] These patients stopped the exogenous estrogen but were randomized in the clinical trials. We do not know what the recurrence rate of stroke would be in someone who stops their estrogen administration.

It is possible that these patients would have a much lower chance of recurrent stroke once estrogen therapy is stopped. If so, their inclusion in the randomized clinical trials would make the recurrence rate much lower in the medical treatment arm and would have diminished the apparent effectiveness of the device arm.

Migraine and Stroke

Another fascinating area is the connection between migraine headaches and stroke. In one study of 1200 ischemic stroke patients, among those who had a stroke of unknown origin, the frequency of PFO was 60%. Of patients who had a stroke of unknown etiology and migraine with frequent aura, the frequency of PFO was 93%.[14] When I was in medical school, the teaching was that the increased frequency of stroke in people with migraine was because migraine was due to transient intense vasoconstriction of the cerebral arteries. The blood vessels then dilated, which caused the throbbing sensation of a migraine. The belief was that if vasoconstriction was strong enough, it would cause the ischemic stroke seen in migraineurs. This theory of migraine is now superseded by experimental data, showing that migraine aura is associated with cortical spreading depolarization. In laboratory studies on transgenic mice that are given the gene for human migraine with hemiplegia, it has been demonstrated that a migraine starts with vasodilation and is then followed by mild vasoconstriction. But the degree of vasoconstriction is about 20% diameter reduction, which is not enough to cause an ischemic brain infarct. The current theory is that migraine is due to a complex interaction within several cortical centers that stimulate nociceptive fibers and receptors responsible for the cephalgia. Migraine is no longer thought of as a "vascular headache," but rather a complex central nervous system event with allodynia.[15]

What is the connection then between migraine and stroke? We believe that stroke is more prevalent in migraineurs because migraine is the clinical manifestation that a large PFO is likely to be present. Fifty percent of people with migraine with aura have a PFO.[16] The PFO conduit permits some vasoactive substance (perhaps serotonin) to bypass metabolism in the lungs and enter the cerebral circulation to trigger a migraine in susceptible people. The migraine identifies those people who are likely to have a PFO pathway, which later in life could permit a venous thrombus to also enter the cerebral circulation. In those migraineurs who also take estrogen compounds, the risk of stroke is even higher because they now have a stimulant for venous thrombosis as well as the PFO pathway to the brain. These considerations have led to the following 2 hypotheses. I believe these to be correct based on my observations and I hope that they will be tested someday in a prospective clinical trial.

- Almost all strokes that occur in young patients with migraine are caused by a paradoxical embolus through a PFO. Migraines do not cause stroke from intense vasospasm; they are the clinical clue that a PFO may be present. Corollary: the increased risk of stroke in migraineurs who take estrogen is due to the more likely presence of a PFO in migraineurs.
- Almost all strokes that occur in young women who take birth control pills are caused by a paradoxical embolus through a PFO. Estrogen does not cause arterial cerebral thrombosis, but rather, predisposes to venous thrombosis which then embolizes through the PFO pathway.

Patent Foramen Ovale and Altitude Sickness

The most enjoyable research project with which I have been involved in my 40 years of academic medicine was our study evaluating the connection between a right-to-left shunt through a PFO and the susceptibility to altitude sickness. This project is described more completely in "PFO and Acute Mountain Sickness". Briefly, to recruit patients who hiked at high altitude, an associate and I backpacked to 12,000 feet on the Mount Whitney trail in the Sierra Nevada, California and stayed at Trail Camp for 1 week. We recruited individuals hiking over Mount Whitney from Whitney Portal in 1 or 2 days and hikers who had acclimated and crossed the John Muir Trail before they climbed Mount Whitney and then exited at Whitney portal. Subjects were referred to the South Inyo Hospital in Lone Pine at the base of the mountain, which graciously permitted us to obtain questionnaires and perform TCD bubble studies in a side room. Hikers who completed the study were given a $25 gift card to spend at the local pizza and beer restaurant in Lone Pine. What ravenously hungry hiker would scoff at that opportunity? We enrolled 137 subjects. The study demonstrated that 63% of hikers who complained of altitude sickness symptoms had a right-to-left shunt.[17] As the oxygen saturation decreases with increasing altitude, hikers with an inherent PFO would be more likely to have right-to-left shunting and desaturate even further than those without a PFO. Anyone attempting to climb Mount Everest or similar heights may wish to consider obtaining a TCD before their ascent (**Figs. 1** and **2**).

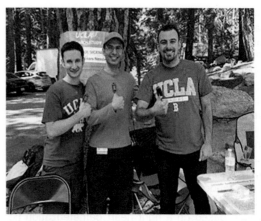

Fig. 1. Brian West, MD (*left*), Pooya Banankhah, MD (*middle*), and Bashar Al Hemyari, MD (*right*) at Whitney Portal to recruit hikers before or after their ascent to Mount Whitney.

Platypnea–Orthodeoxia and Patent Foramen Ovale

Another fascinating condition associated with PFO is unexpected profound hypoxemia, often with sudden onset such as following surgery, in people who have dilatation or uncoiling of the aorta or other thoracic abnormalities such as pulmonary lobectomy or hemidiaphragm paralysis. These people have no dyspnea and normal arterial saturation when they lie supine but become short of breath and desaturate to 75% to 85% oxygen saturation as soon as they stand up. It is often difficult to make this diagnosis unless you are thinking about it in your differential for hypoxemia out of proportion to the amount of pulmonary disease (if any), but the patients are completely relieved of their orthodeoxia and shortness of breath after the PFO is closed.[18,19] Using TEE, we have demonstrated that the PFO height between the septum primum

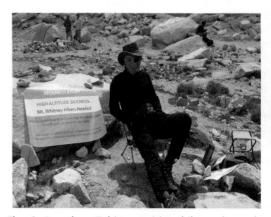

Fig. 2. Jonathan Tobis recruiting hikers along the John Muir Trail at 12,000′ Trail Camp.

and secundum is wider in the upright position when compared with the supine position (Tobis and Yang, unpublished data).

Sleep Apnea and Patent Foramen Ovale

Another area of significant clinical hypoxemia that is associated with PFO is in people who have sleep apnea. PFO occurs in a higher frequency of patients who have obstructive sleep apnea. In one study of 100 patients with sleep apnea, the frequency of PFO was 43% versus the control population of 200 individuals where the incidence of PFO was 20% (P<.02).[20] There are other reports of sleep apnea patients with a PFO who have significant improvement in their hypoxemia and clinical symptoms of sleep apnea after their PFO is closed.[21] This topic should be addressed in a prospective randomized double-blinded clinical trial of PFO closure in patients who have sleep apnea with a PFO.

Coronary Artery Spasm and Patent Foramen Ovale

A last topic that I would like to touch upon is a recently described syndrome of severe chest pain plus migraine (usually with aura), in women who have a PFO. I have seen 10 patients like this, which is a rare occurrence for people with PFO, but we have documented angiographic evidence of coronary artery spasm with an abnormal response to intracoronary acetylcholine. These women have recurrent episodes of severe angina-like chest pain which can occur intermittently over several years. This condition is not benign; two of the patients had an episode of ventricular fibrillation associated with severe chest pain from which they was resuscitated. All had a PFO and in those 7 who had their PFO closed, both chest pain and migraine symptoms resolved.[22] We believe that there is some vasoactive substance which normally gets detoxified in passage through the pulmonary circulation, but when exposed to the arterial blood in high concentration, can induce coronary spasm and/or migraine in susceptible individuals. It is my hope that those researchers who are currently studying Ischemia with Non Obstructive Coronary Arteries (INOCA) (myocardial ischemia with no obstructive coronary arteries) will also assess the frequency of PFO in this unusual population of coronary spasm or microvascular ischemia (**Figs. 3** and **4**).

Complications of Patent Foramen Ovale Closure

With improved occluder devices available today and techniques standardized, the complication

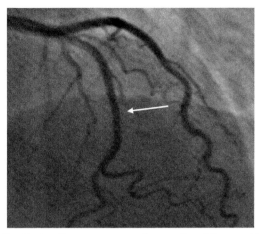

Fig. 3. Baseline coronary angiogram in a 68 year old woman with angina symptoms at rest, migraines, and a PFO. The *white arrow* identifies the Left Anterior Descending artery.

rate of percutaneous PFO closure should be close to zero, making it the safest therapeutic interventional cardiology procedure. Bleeding from the femoral vein can be reduced by placing a Perclose suture prior to insertion of the 11-French sheath. However, there are 2 complications that are worthy of comment.

Atrial Fibrillation Following Patent Foramen Ovale Closure

There is an increased incidence of new-onset atrial fibrillation (AF) after a closure device is placed across the atrial septum. It is believed that this is due to the pressure applied to the interatrial tissue and the presence of a foreign body in the heart. Post-closure AF appears to be relatively benign

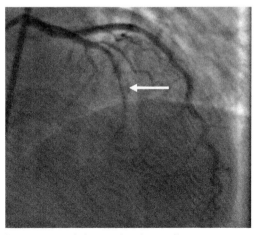

Fig. 4. Intense left anterior descending artery spasm after intracoronary administration of 100 μg acetylcholine. The *white arrow* identies the same location as in the baseline picture.

and usually does not need long-term anticoagulation since it is not associated with recurrent stroke. However, the symptoms of tachycardia and chest thumping are uncomfortable for the patient and produces anxiety unless they are forewarned of this possibility. To prevent thrombus forming in the left atrium, I treat post-closure AF with short-term apixaban and amiodarone for 6 to 8 weeks. There is no standard therapy and other operators have a variety of approaches. The good news is that the AF is intermittent and transient, always resolving spontaneously. Onset of AF is typically 10 to 14 days post-device closure and it dissipates within 1 month of onset. In our series of 445 patients, older age was not a predictor of developing AF, but male sex was.[23] The REDUCE trial also found male sex to be an independent predictor of postprocedural AF in patients who underwent closure with either Gore Cardioform or Helex devices (OR = 3.45, $P < .01$).[24] The rate of AF is approximately 4% with the Amplatzer PFO device but is 16% for the Cardioform occluder, presumably due to greater pressure exerted on the septum with the Gore device. The trade-off is that the complete closure rate with the Cardioform device is 98%, whereas the Amplatzer PFO device has a 15% incidence of residual shunting.[25]

Need for Surgical Removal of the Device

The second potential complication with PFO closure is significant, but fortunately rare. About 1 in 500 cases develop some complication with the device or the patient has such severe chest pain that surgical removal is required. The mechanism appears slightly different for the 2 major devices. The Amplatzer device seems to leach more nickel from the nitinol wires. Since 12% of people are allergic to nickel, it should be expected that some might react to this product.[26] In a survey of close to 14,000 cases around the world, the reported need for surgical removal was 0.2% for either the Amplatzer or the Cardioform device.[27] The Amplatzer atrial septal defect (ASD) or PFO device can erode the atrial wall and the Cardioform nitinol wires may fracture and rarely, perforate the heart causing hemopericardium.[28] This low risk appears justified if the indication for closure was to prevent recurrent stroke. However, if closure for migraine is approved by the Food and Drug Administration, then we will be placing these devices in younger patients. There is still room for clever bioengineers to develop devices that are as effective as the current ones, but without the need for any surgical removal.

We hope you enjoy reading the chapters presented in this edition of Clinics in Cardiology that explore the broad clinical spectrum of this residual embryologic cardiac defect called PFO.

CLINICS CARE POINTS

- The echocardiographic criteria for the diagnosis and sizing of a patent foramen ovale (PFO) need to be updated by the appropriate society's guideline committees. Echocardiography underestimates the size of a PFO and the statement on the echo reports that there is "a small PFO" should not be interpreted as "this PFO is too small to cause a stroke."

- Similarly, the late appearance of bubbles in the left atrium does not mean that there is a transpulmonary shunt or pulmonary arteriovenous malformation; 99 times out of 100, late bubbles are due to a PFO.

- I believe that the following hypotheses will eventually be proven to be correct:

  Hypothesis #1

  Almost all strokes that occur in young patients with migraine are caused by a paradoxic embolus through a PFO. Migraines do not cause stroke from intense vasospasm; they are the clinical clue that a PFO may be present.

  Corollary: the increased risk of stroke in migraineurs who take estrogen is due to the more likely presence of a PFO in migraineurs.

- Hypothesis #2

  Almost all strokes that occur in young women who take birth control pills are caused by a paradoxic embolus through a PFO. Estrogen does not cause arterial cerebral thrombosis, but rather, predisposes to venous thrombosis which then embolizes through the PFO pathway.

- Unexplained hypoxemia, especially after surgery, may be due to severe right-to-left shunting through a PFO. The clinician has to consider this possibility and then look for it with the appropriate test of an agitated saline bubble study, of which a transcranial Doppler is the most sensitive test and therefore the preferred screening modality.

- Angina with No Obstructive Coronary Arteries (ANOCA) with documented coronary artery spasm may be associated with a PFO. The right-to-left shunt of vasoactive substances may precipitate coronary artery spasm in susceptible people. Unless one looks for the right-to-left shunt, you will never know if it is there and that it could be causally related.

DISCLOSURE

Dr J.M. Tobis is a consultant and proctor for WL Gore, Inc.

REFERENCES

1. Elgendy A, Saver J, Tobis JM, et al. Proposal for updated nomenclature and classification of potential Causative mechanism in patent foramen ovale–associated stroke. JAMA Neurol 2020;77(7):878–86.

2. Kent DM, Saver JL, Kasner SE, et al. Heterogeneity of treatment Effects in an analysis of pooled individual patient data from randomized trials of device closure of patent foramen ovale after stroke. JAMA 2021;326(22).

3. Mahmoud AN, Elgendy IY, Agarwal N, et al. Identification and Quantification of patent foramen ovale-Mediated shunts: echocardiography and transcranial Doppler. Interv Cardiol Clin 2017;6(4):495–504.

4. Mojadidi MK, Mahmoud AN, Elgendy IY, et al. Transesophageal echocardiography for the detection of patent foramen ovale. J Am Soc Echocardiogr 2017;30(9):933–4.

5. Mojadidi MK, Zhang L, Chugh Y, et al. Transcranial Doppler: does addition of blood to agitated saline Affect Sensitivity for Detecting cardiac right-to-left shunt? Echocardiography 2016;33(8):1219–27.

6. Mojadidi MK, Winoker JS, Roberts SC, et al. Accuracy of Conventional transthoracic echocardiography for the diagnosis of Intracardiac right-to-left shunt: a meta-analysis of prospective studies. Echocardiography 2014;31(9):1036–48.

7. Mojadidi MK, Bogush N, Caceres JD, et al. Diagnostic accuracy of transesophageal echocardiogram for the detection of patent foramen ovale: a meta-analysis. Echocardiography 2014;31(6):752–8.

8. Gevorgyan R, Perlowski A, Shenoda M, et al. Sensitivity of Brachial versus femoral vein injection of agitated saline to Detect right-to-left shunts with transcranial Doppler. Catheter Cardiovasc Interv 2014. https://doi.org/10.1002/ccd.25391.

9. Turc G, Lee J-Y, Brochet E, et al, on behalf of the CLOSE and DEFENSE-PFO Trial Investigators. Atrial aneurysm, ShuntSize, and recurrent stroke risk in patients with patent foramen ovale. J Am Coll Cardiol 2020;75(18):2312–20.

10. Kijima Y, Gevorgyan R, McWilliams JP, et al. Usefulness of transcranial Doppler for Detecting pulmonary Arteriovenous malformations in hereditary hemorrhagic telangiectasia. Am J Cardiology 2016;117(7):1180–4.

11. Saver JL, Carroll JD, Thaler DE, et al. For the RESPECT Investigators* long-term Outcomes of patent foramen ovale closure or medical therapy after stroke. N Engl J Med 2017;377.

12. Greep NC, Liebeskind DS, Gevorgyan R, et al. Association of ischemic stroke, hormone therapy, and right to left shunt in Postmenopausal women. Catheter Cardiovasc Interv 2014;84(3):479–85.

13. Subrata Kar DO, Nabil Noureddin MD, Jamil Aboulhosn MD, et al. Percutaneous closure of patent foramen ovale or atrial septal defect in the presence of thrombophilia. Journal of Structural Heart Disease 2017;3(5):135–40.

14. West BH, Noureddin N, Mamzhi Y, et al. Frequency of patent foramen ovale and migraine in patients with cryptogenic stroke. Stroke 2018;49(5):1123–8.

15. Charles A, Hansen J. Migraine aura: new ideas about cause, classification, and clinical significance. Curr Opin Neurol 2015;28(3):255–60.

16. Anzola G. Potential Source of cerebral embolism in migraine with aura: a transcranial Doppler study. Neurology 1999;52(8):1622–5.

17. West BH, Fleming RG, Al Hemyari B, et al. Relation of patent foramen ovale to Acute mountain sickness. Am J Cardiol 2019;123(12):2022–5.

18. Tobis JM, Abudayyeh I. Platypnea-orthodeoxia syndrome: an Overlooked cause of hypoxemia. JACC Cardiovasc Interv 2016;9(18):1939–40.

19. Mojadidi MK, Gevorgyan R, Noureddin N, et al. The effect of patent foramen ovale closure in patients with platypnea-orthodeoxia syndrome. Cathet Cardiovasc Interv 2015;86(4):701–7.

20. Mojadidi MK, Bokhoor PI, Gevorgyan R, et al. Sleep apnea in patients with and without a right-to-left shunt. J. Clin Sleep Medicine 2015;11(11):1299–304.

21. White JM, Veale AG, Ruygrok PN. Patent foramen ovale closure in the treatment of obstructive sleep apnea. J Invasive Cardiol 2013;25:E169–71.

22. Ravi D, Parikh R, Aboulhosn J, Tobis JM. A new syndrome of patent foramen ovale inducing Vasospastic angina and migraine. JACC Case Reports 2023;28:102132.

23. Incidence of Atrial Fibrillation or Arrhythmias After Patent Foramen Ovale Closure Keeley Ravellette, Jeff Gornbein, Jonathan M. Tobis; JSCAI 2023.

24. Søndergaard L, Kasner SE, Rhodes JF, et al. Patent foramen ovale closure or Antiplatelet therapy for cryptogenic stroke. N Engl J Med 2017;377:1033–42.

25. Matsumura K, Gevorgyan R, Mangols D, et al. Comparison of residual shunt rates in five devices used to treat patent foramen ovale. Catheter Cardiovasc Interv 2014;84(3):455–63.

26. Brett Wertman MD, Babak Azarbal MD, Marc Riedl MD, et al. Adverse events associated with nickel Allergy in patients Undergoing percutaneous ASD or PFO closure. J Am Coll Cardiol 2006;47(6):1226–7.

27. Verma SK, Tobis JM. Explantation of PFO closure devices: a Multicenter survey. JACC Cardiovasc Interv 2011;4(5):579–85.

28. Kumar P, Orford J, Tobis JM. Two cases of pericardial tamponade due to nitinol wire fracture of a gore septal occluder. Catheter Cardiovasc Interv 2019;1–6.

Patent Foramen Ovale Embryology, Anatomy, and Physiology

Adeba Mohammad, DO, MS[a], HuuTam Truong, MD, FSCAI[b], Islam Abudayyeh, MD, MPH, FSCAI[c],*

KEYWORDS

- Patent foramen ovale • Transesophageal echocardiography • Intracardiac echocardiography
- Anatomy • Physiology • Embryology • Septum primum • Septum secundum

KEY POINTS

- The foramen ovale is formed as part of the normal embryologic development but remains patent in 20% to 25% of adults due to incomplete fusion of the septum primum and septum secundum.
- Right-to-left shunting from a patent foramen ovale (PFO) is often clinically silent but may become pathologic when associated with other conditions such as venous thrombosis and elevated right-sided pressures.
- The anatomy of PFO varies in complexity with different characteristics such as diameter, tunnel length, aneurysm, and thickness necessitating thorough investigation prior to closure.

INTRODUCTION

Detailed familiarity with interatrial septal anatomy and the surrounding structures is essential to understand the physiology of patent foramen ovale (PFO) and possible septal pathology. Knowledge of atrial septal anatomy is also important to safely perform interventions through the septum and in the process of closing septal defects. To describe the anatomy, this article will begin by presenting the embryology of the atrial septal formation and how surrounding structures are influenced during development to reach the mature form. Presenting the structure of the interatrial septum and foramen ovale from the standpoint of different imaging modalities provides a more complete appreciation of the anatomy as it appears to a proceduralist. A consideration of hemodynamics and the patient's clinical condition that can influence PFO physiology provides a comprehensive clinical picture and aids in decision-making.

PATENT FORAMEN OVALE EMBRYOLOGY

The formation of bilateral atria and the foramen ovale begins at 4 weeks of embryo development.[1,2] The septum primum divides the primitive atria into a right and left atrium. The septum primum is a muscular structure with a mesenchymal cap at the leading edge that grows from the primitive atrial roof toward the inferior and superior endocardial cushions, leaving a crescent-shaped large opening connecting the atria known as the ostium primum. The endocardial cushions grow from ventral and dorsal aspects of the atrioventricular (AV) canal until they fuse, resulting in the division of AV canal into right and left sides and form the right and left channels which constitute the primitive AV valves. The septum primum continues to grow toward the fused endocardial cushions, decreasing the size of the ostium primum until it completely disappears. Simultaneously, perforations are formed more proximally in the superior

---

[a] Cardiology Department, Loma Linda University Health, 1234 Anderson Street, Loma Linda, CA 92354, USA; [b] VA Loma Linda Healthcare System, 11201 Benton Street, Loma Linda, CA 92354, USA; [c] VA Loma Linda Healthcare System, Charles Drew University, 11201 Benton Street, Loma Linda, CA 92354, USA
* Corresponding author.
E-mail address: iabudayyeh@mac.com

Cardiol Clin 42 (2024) 463–472
https://doi.org/10.1016/j.ccl.2024.01.004
0733-8651/24/Published by Elsevier Inc.

septum primum via programmed cell death, creating an ostium (foramen) secundum. **Fig. 1**.

Blood is then shunted in utero from the right atrium (RA) to the left atrium via the foramen secundum. The septum secundum is a crescent-shaped membrane that develops in the 12th week of fetal development from the ventrocranial atrial wall to the right of the septum primum, partially covering the foramen secundum, leaving a window opening inferiorly known as the foramen ovale. The septum primum forms a flaplike valve over the foramen ovale. The critical function of the foramen ovale is to allow shunting of oxygenated blood from the placenta via the umbilical vein and inferior vena cava (IVC) to the systemic circulation. The sinus venosus forms the superior vena cava (SVC) and IVC. The Chiari network shunts blood from the IVC directly toward the septum secundum into the foramen ovale, thus directing oxygenated blood into the left atrium and systemic circulation. The SVC directs deoxygenated blood downward toward the tricuspid valve into the right heart and pulmonary circulation. The foramen ovale shunting of oxygenated blood is necessary since during fetal development, the lungs are filled with amniotic fluid and do not function to oxygenate blood. To deliver oxygenated blood from the umbilical vein to critical organs, the blood is shunted through the foramen ovale into the left atrium as well as across the ductus arteriosus from the pulmonary artery into the descending aorta. Placental blood has limited oxygen at 67% saturation. If the placental blood were directed through the nonoxygenating fetal pulmonary circulation, it would continue to lose oxygen and thus be insufficient to oxygenate the fetal organs. This mechanism of supplying oxygenated blood to the fetus is so essential that it is preserved throughout evolution such that all mammals have a PFO.

At birth, there is an acute drop in pulmonary pressure and right atrial pressure, with expulsion of fluid from the lungs, resulting in the left atrial pressure exceeding the right atrial pressure. This change in atrial pressures results in closure of the septum primum on the septum secundum and the newly closed section of the atrial septum is called the fossa ovale. In approximately 4 out of 5 adults, the tissue of the septum primum is fused to the septum secundum and the interatrial tunnel in the fossa ovale is sealed. However, in 20% to 25% of people, the tissue of the septum primum does not fuse with the septum secundum and the remaining flap of the septum primum remains open and is known as a PFO.[3] Transient changes in right-sided pressures and flow from the IVC directed by the residual eustachian valve will allow some deoxygenated venous blood to crossover into the left atrium. This flow may carry blood clots and gas bubbles, or chemical products that may cause clinically relevant outcomes in the systemic circulation.

ANATOMY

The interatrial septum is angled in the long axis of the patient, from the posterior right to the anterior left with the left atrium being the most posterior structure of the heart and the RA on the right just over the spine. Therefore, the atrial septum is anatomically tilted at an oblique angle toward the RA, bringing the foramen ovale superior and in-line with the IVC flow into the RA. **Fig. 2**.

From the operator's standpoint, the left atrium is posterior against the esophagus, while the RA is anterior and to the patient's right. **Fig. 3**.

Understanding this anatomic arrangement allows the operator to appreciate the septum and surrounding anatomy during septal interventions using different modalities such as transesophageal echocardiography (TEE), intracardiac echocardiography (ICE), and fluoroscopy.

Multiple factors affect the physiologic tilt of the septum, including the patient's age, body habitus, and size and shape of the heart and its chambers. Usually, younger, lean patients with vertical hearts without enlarged chambers have less tilt compared to patients who are obese with more horizontal hearts. Similarly, right atrial enlargement will push the right ventricle (RV) anteriorly against the chest wall and inferiorly toward the diaphragm as the RV is constrained by the interventricular septum such that the tricuspid valve becomes vertical and can enhance the direction of flow from the IVC toward the atrial septum.

Implication of Interatrial Septum During Transseptal Puncture

Because of the oblique orientation of the septum, some trans-septal punctures via the femoral vein approach end up occurring near the superior rim of the fossa ovale since the needle tends to slip slightly superiorly when force is applied.[4] Furthermore, the less oblique the septum is, the more difficult it is to perform trans-septal punctures. In such patients, a curve on the needle along with gentle traction on the hub helps avoid superior slip during the septal puncture. When encountering a highly mobile or thick septum, radiofrequency-assisted puncture by use of a cutting Bovie or a specific radiofrequency needle can allow safer septal crossing without the need to apply undue force and risk the needle slipping.[5] To perform a trans-septal puncture, the operator

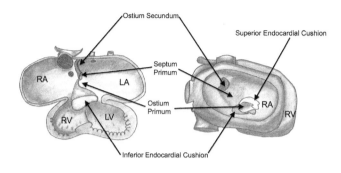

Fig. 1. Embryologic representation of atrial septal development from the first to the third trimester. The overlap of the septum secundum and primum primum creates the fossa ovale and, if not sealed shortly after birth, the patent foramen ovale develops. (*Courtesy* Dr. Payush Chatta.)

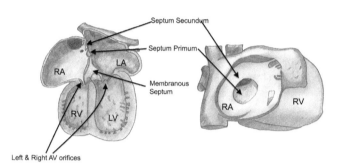

begins with the sheath and needle in the SVC and with some clockwise torque and traction pulls the sheath back without exposing the needle. There should be 2 discrete rightward "drops" as the sheath first drops into the RA from the SVC and then drops into the fossa ovale. The clockwise torque maintains the direction of the access sheath posterior which, as discussed earlier, is the en face aspect of the interatrial septum. **Fig. 4.**

In approximately 20% to 34% of people, the septa do not fuse resulting in a PFO.[6] In this scenario, the septum secundum and retro-aortic rim form the superior and anterior rims of the fossa. The septum primum overlaps the opening from the left atrial side. The slightly higher left atrial pressure maintains the septum primum against the rims keeping the fossa closed. On occasion, due to a transient rise in right-sided pressures such as with a Valsalva maneuver or coughing, it is possible for the mobile septum primum to be pushed back allowing non-hemodynamically significant flow from the RA to the left atrium. **Fig. 5.**

Due to the high prevalence of PFO in the general population, right-to-left shunting can have significant clinical outcomes if emboli cross into the systemic circulation. PFOs vary in shape, size, and mobility. From autopsy studies, PFOs range in diameter from a mean of 3.4 mm during first decade of life to 5.8 mm in diameter in the ninth decade of life, with larger diameters being more common in women than men.[7,8] The length of overlap between the septum primum and septum secundum determines the PFO length, which can present as a tunnel-like passage. The tunnel lengths can range from 5 mm to 13 mm.[9] PFOs are characterized as simple or complex. Features of complex PFO include tunnel length greater than 10 mm, PFO with a septal aneurysm, multiple openings of PFO on left atrial side, association with Eustachian valve or ridge, excessive hypertrophy of septum secundum, or association with additional defects (such as atrial septal defect

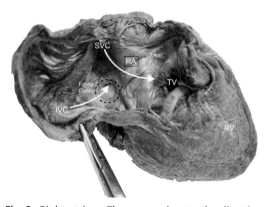

Fig. 2. Right atrium. The arrows denote the direction of blood return into the right atrium. The inferior vena cava (IVC) directs blood toward the septum and the PFO while the superior vena cava (SVC) directs blood toward the tricuspid valve (TV).

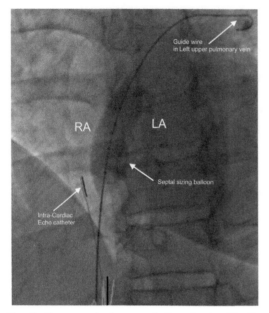

Fig. 3. Fluoroscopic image of the chest with the guidewire in the left upper pulmonary vein and sizing balloon across the atrial septum. Guidance is by use of intracardiac echocardiography (ICE). Waist in the balloon shows the area where the septum partially constrains the balloon at the level separating the right atrium (RA) and left atrium (LA).

[ASD]) (**Table 1**).[10] On occasion, a hand injection of angiographic contrast during the procedure can provide additional information about the location and geometry of the PFO. Using a sizing balloon at the time of cardiac catheterization can help size the PFO tunnel and provide guidance in choosing the appropriate occluder size.

Detailed knowledge of the individual PFO anatomy is important for safe closure and allows the operator to anticipate challenges based on the characteristics described. Septum primum

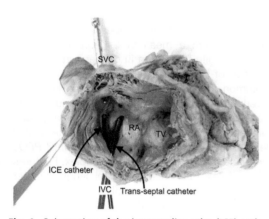

Fig. 4. Orientation of the intracardiac echo (ICE) catheter and trans-septal sheaths as they enter the right atrium via the inferior vena cava (IVC).

aneurysm occasionally exists, which is defined as a septal deflection from the neutral atrial septum plane into either the atrium greater than 10 mm or a total greater than 15 mm into both chambers. The prevalence of atrial septal aneurysm as per autopsy studies in the general population is 2% to 3%.[11] PFO is associated with atrial septal aneurysm between 6.9% and greater than 50%.[12–14] The variation of the incidence of PFO in reports appears to be related to the sensitivity of the technique for identifying a right-to-left shunt. In the authors' experience with 600 PFO closures, the authors have almost always found a PFO when there is an atrial septal aneurysm. Septal aneurysms can also affect PFO closure. The ideal way to study PFO anatomy is via a TEE, whereby the septum can be visualized in 3 dimensions. Using TEE, the best view to visualize the atrial septum is the bicaval view at omniplane angle 100 to 140° with right rotation of the probe. Here, the left atrium will be at the top of the screen and the RA on the bottom, with SVC and IVC to the right and left, respectively. Alternatively, ICE can be used during a clinical procedure with the probe in the RA facing the septum. Using ICE, the RA will be on top of the screen, and IVC and SVC will be to the left and right, respectively. Rotating the ICE screen image 90° counterclockwise, the ICE image will appear in the same anatomic orientation as fluoroscopy.[15,16]

By definition, a PFO has an intact atrial rim. Any missing part of the septum allows a permanent communication between the atria and is termed an ASD.

IMAGING ANATOMY

For safe and successful closure of a PFO, operators use different imaging modalities to guide the procedure. The most common modalities are TEE, ICE, and fluoroscopy. Knowledge of how to obtain appropriate images of the atrial and septal structures from each of these modalities is helpful to understand how the images present the anatomy. This conceptual analysis of how the 2-dimensional images demonstrate the 3-dimensional anatomy helps the interventionist to form a more complete overall picture.

FLUOROSCOPY DURING PATENT FORAMEN OVALE CLOSURE

With the x-ray fluoroscopy system in the anteroposterior-view, a wire is advanced typically from the IVC approach which appears just left of the spine on the screen (right of the patient's spine). The wire then should cross the septum

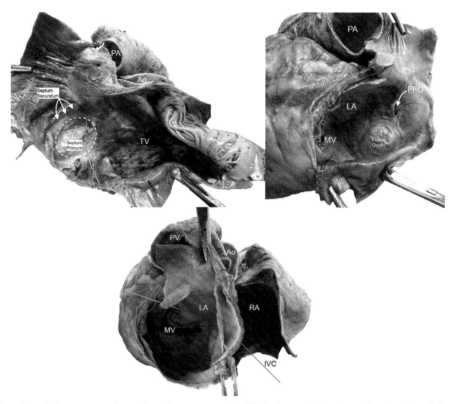

Fig. 5. Direction of flow across the patent foramen ovale (PFO) denoted by the teal string. Top left: From the right atrial side, the flow travels along the septum primum and enters the left atrium (LA) posteriorly to the septum secundum. Top right: The flow from the PFO is directed vertically toward the left atrial roof. Bottom: the string demonstrates the direction of flow from the right atrium (RA) through the PFO and into the LA as well as the approximate angle.

overlaying the spine and to the top left of the patient's chest. Care must be applied when advancing the wire to avoid the left atrial appendage (LAA) and to try to position the J-tip in the left upper pulmonary vein. This appears on the screen as the tip of the wire outside of the cardiac silhouette and is confirmed by echocardiography, as described in the following paragraphs. It is also possible to place the wire in the right upper pulmonary vein where the wire takes a more midline course and then to the right of the chest where it exits the cardiac silhouette. Should the operator note any bending or resistance on the wire, they should stop and check the wire position by echocardiography. The LAA is trabeculated with varying thickness based on location. The greatest thickness is anterior (3.2 ± 1.4 mm) followed by superior (2.5 ± 1.0 mm), inferior (2.2 ± 0.8 mm), and posterior (2.2 ± 0.8 mm). Therefore, the LAA is vulnerable to perforation especially if a stiff or straight-tipped wire is used.[17] When using a sizing balloon to judge PFO tunnel length, height, and width, or to modify the PFO to better accept the closure device, the

balloon is positioned primarily over the spine and the waist should overlap the mid-line. A steep left anterior oblique (LAO)-cranial angulation (approximately 35° LAO and 15° cranial) allows the operator to see along the plane of the septum separating the right and left atria and device deployment in profile. Device position and septal capture are all best visualized in that view. Once the device is deployed a right anterior oblique-caudal view shows the device en face. While this view is not as important, the operator can visualize the fully expanded disc and if it had been constrained or misshaped by the tunnel.

RADIATION EXPOSURE CONSIDERATIONS

Unlike echocardiography that does not produce appreciable energy exposure, fluoroscopy uses X-rays to produce an image. Structural anatomy and PFOs are much larger than coronary vessels and do not require the level of detail typically demanded during precise coronary interventions. Therefore, the authors recommend lowering the radiation exposure as much as possible as the

Table 1
Characteristics of complex patent foramen ovale anatomy

Complex PFO Characteristics:	
Tunnel length	>10 mm in length
Aneurysmal septum	>10 mm unidirectional deflection or>15 mm bidirectionally
Thick or lipomatous septum secundum	>10 mm in thickness
Multiple defects	Multi-fenestrated septum or associated with small ASDs
Access and cardiac confounders:	
Prominent Eustachian valve or Chiari network	Can make crossing into the RA and directing devices across the septum more challenging
Distorted, shortened, or rotated aortic root and septal anatomy	Difficulty visualizing the anatomy by ICE and deploying the closure devices perpendicular to the defect

Abbreviations: ASDs, atrial septal defect; ICE, intracardiac echocardiography; PFO, patent foramen ovale; RA, right atrium.

operators should be able to visualize all pertinent structures, wires, and closure devices without difficulty. This is especially important when operating on younger patients at higher risk from radiation exposure sequelae.

TRANSESOPHAGEAL ECHOCARDIOGRAPHY

Since the esophagus is a posterior structure and adjacent to the spine, the transesophageal probe produces images of the heart where the most proximal structure is the left atrium. The higher frequency of a TEE probe provides higher spatial resolution to produce detailed rendering of the left atrium and left side of the septum. With the probe in the low esophageal plane, the operator will see the AV valves along with the inferior-anterior segment of the interatrial septum. To see the tricuspid valve, the operator rotates the TEE probe clockwise from the mitral view or changes the omniplane angle. Pulling the TEE probe back shows more of the septum and, once the aortic root is in the short axis view, the operator can scan across the septum from the anterior-superior retro-aortic segment posteriorly to the fossa ovale at the junction of the septum primum and septum secundum. This is done by rotating the TEE probe counterclockwise to point the imaging component posteriorly and by rotating the omniplane to show different aspects of the septum and surrounding anatomy. **Fig. 6**.

The retro-aortic area adjacent to the aorta is the most commonly deficient rim in atrial septum secundum defects but should be intact in PFOs. Rotating the probe more posteriorly demonstrates the superior aspect of the septum secundum.

INTRACARDIAC ECHOCARDIOGRAPHY

ICE imaging allows the operator to manage the imaging component without an echocardiographer or an anesthesiology team. As the probe is in the RA, it directly images the interatrial septum from the right side. The typical ICE imaging catheter functions at between 5 and 10 MHz. This is in contrast to TEE which images at 6 to 7 Mhz and transthoracic echocardiography at 2 to 4 Mhz. The higher frequency provides more detailed images but with lower penetration. As the ICE probe is in the RA, the top structure on the screen (structure closest to the probe) is the RA, which is the converse of a TEE image. From the home view and with the ICE catheter neutral of deflection, the operator would see the RA at the top, RV at

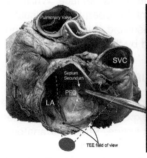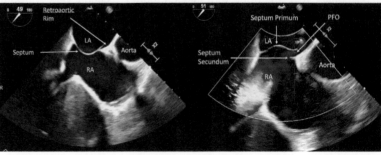

Fig. 6. Left: Gross anatomy of the left atrium (LA) with the location of the transesophageal probe (TEE) and its field of view. Right: TEE-generated images showing the aorta, retro-aortic rim, septum secundum, and septum primum. The left atrium is closest to the probe (top of echo imaging) since the esophagus lays directly posterior to it with the right atrium (RA) on the other side of the septum.

the bottom with the tricuspid valve between. Rotating the probe clockwise and with posterior tilt on the probe brings the aorta into view. Once the aorta is in position, further clockwise rotation moves the imaging beam posteriorly to scan the septum anteriorly from the aorta to the SVC posteriorly. Midway between the aorta and the vena cava is the fossa ovale. Minimal right and left tilt with minimal clockwise rotation will show all aspects of the fossa ovale. The interatrial septum appears horizontally across the screen. The septum secundum is on the right side of the screen and the septum primum on the left. The 2 structures are easily distinguished because the septum primum is thin (1–2.5 mm) compared with the thicker septum secundum (4-9 mm).[18] In some cases, it is not possible to see all the aspects of the septum primum well due to thinness or mobility. Applying color flow allows the operator to better understand the septal shape and mobility as well as screen for small fenestrated defects especially in aneurysmal anatomy.

With minimal manipulation, the operator is then able to visualize the left atrium and LAA at the 4 to 6 o'clock position with the left atrium at the bottom of the screen. This view is helpful when advancing the wire into the left atrium across the septum so as to avoid placing the wire in the LAA. Further rotation of the probe clockwise brings into view the pulmonary veins, the more favorable structures in which to place the guidewire, and finally, more posteriorly, the SVC. It is not always possible to visualize the IVC with ICE due to its position as it enters the RA, but the operator may be able to see the Eustachian valve at the IVC-RA junction. **Fig. 7**.

HEMODYNAMICS

A PFO is usually clinically silent as left-to-right shunting across the foramen ovale when patent does not produce enough volume loading on the RV to cause structural heart changes. This is in contrast to larger secundum ASDs which do induce structural changes in the heart if the ASD is more than 1 cm in diameter. As such, assessments of the pulmonary to systemic flow (Qp:Qs) are not typically done for the assessment of PFO. However, in a subgroup of patients, small transient right to left flow across the septum may produce clinically relevant complications including platypnea orthodeoxia, emboli causing stroke, myocardial infarction, decompression illness and other systemic vascular injuries. Factors that promote right-to-left shunting include septal anatomy such as a mobile or aneurysmal septum; patient factors such as high right-sided pressures, venous

thrombosis, pacemaker leads, or catheters across the tricuspid valve; and disorders that acutely affect flow into the right side of the heart. Such disorders include pulmonary infarcts, pulmonary emboli, pneumothorax, rise in pulmonary pressures due to left heart or valve disease, abdominal surgery or insufflation, pneumonectomy, and thoracic interventions. These conditions can all influence the right-sided pressures and direction of the blood entering the RA. Closure of a PFO is usually performed as a response to incidents such as an MRI or computed tomography documentation of stroke or systemic emboli causing ischemia to the heart or other organs.

Platypnea orthodeoxia is a condition where the oxygen saturation is normal when supine but drops below 92% upon sitting up or standing. The mechanism is believed to be due to an increase in right-to-left shunting of venous blood in the upright position. The returning venous blood from the IVC is directed to the PFO tunnel. In addition, there is unpublished TEE evidence that the PFO flap separates from the septum secundum when going from the supine to upright posture in these patients. This enlarges the size of the PFO and permits deoxygenated blood to flow directly to the left atrium. It is distinguished from other causes of hypoxemia by being unresponsive to oxygen supplementation with normal lung function. There is a fairly rapid drop in oxygen saturation when assuming an upright posture and rapid recovery when the patient returns to a supine position.

Decompression sickness (DCS) may occur in scuba divers especially when there is a rapid change in external pressure when ascending. The higher pressure at greater depths permits nitrogen to stay in solution in the body tissues. When the diver ascends, the pressure decrease permits the nitrogen to form bubbles which enter the venous system. If a PFO is present, it is more likely for these nitrogen bubbles to enter the systemic circulation and occlude small arterioles. DCS may have global effects such as fatigue, a skin rash, muscle pain, and joint pain but it can also have detrimental outcomes when a large volume of nitrogen bubbles cross into the systemic circulation and act similar to blood clots in occluding flow through arterioles. As such, patients who have high-risk occupations such as professional deep-sea divers, navy divers, high-altitude pilots, or unpressurized air travel such as in the aerospace field may require prophylactic closure of PFOs.

Due to the anatomic considerations mentioned earlier, agitated saline bubble studies with transthoracic echocardiography have a limited

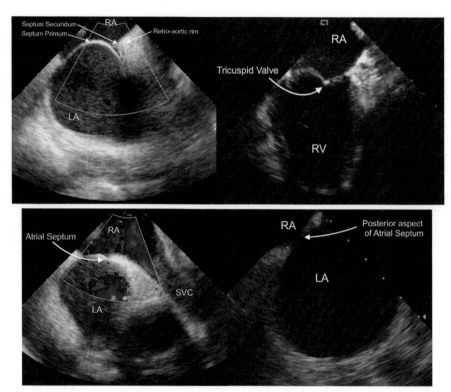

Fig. 7. Top right: Home view or the first view the intracardiac echo (ICE) imaging probe produces in the right atrium (RA). Top left: Clockwise rotation of the probe will bring into view the aorta and retro-aortic rim. Gentle manipulation here to the right will likely show the patent foramen ovale (PFO) tunnel. Bottom right: Further clockwise rotation of the ICE probe will bring into view the posterior aspect of the septum away from the retro-aortic rim. Bottom left: Further clockwise rotation will show the superior vena cava (SVC) and the most posterior aspect of the septum. Note flow from the SVC entering the RA in red.

sensitivity to detect PFOs as low as 50% to 88% depending on the study and analysis.[19–21] Agitated saline bubbles are typically injected through an intravenous catheter placed in the arm. The arm delivers blood to the SVC which directs flow across the tricuspid valve, not toward the PFO. A more effective, if less convenient, approach is to inject the bubbles from the leg so that the flow arrives into the RA through the IVC and is directed by the Eustachian valve toward the foramen ovale.

When performing a septal closure procedure, the bubble study can be performed by injection through the femoral vein catheter under echocardiographic imaging and either with Valsalva or abdominal compression. This allows the operator to appreciate the location of the PFO, magnitude of the shunt, and length of the tunnel. It should also be used to judge if there is another cause for the right-to-left shunting such as a pulmonary arterio-venous malformation (AVM). While less common, large pulmonary AVMs can allow large emboli (2-4 mm) to cross through the pulmonary

circulation and produce systemic embolization. It may be difficult to distinguish a PFO versus a pulmonary AVM by transthoracic echocardiography or even TEE with bubble studies, although imaging bubbles in the pulmonary veins is diagnostic. The pulmonary shunt may be diagnosed by performing the agitated saline bubble study through a catheter that is placed in the pulmonary artery, thereby bypassing the influence of a PFO. If a pulmonary AVM is not present, the agitated saline bubbles injected into the pulmonary artery will be exhaled and no bubbles will be visualized in the left atrium. If a pulmonary AVM is present, the bubbles transfer through the pulmonary AVM and enter the left atrium via the affected pulmonary vein. It is also possible to have both a PFO and a pulmonary AVM.

Imaging During Patent Foramen Ovale Closure

Prior to selecting and deploying the closure device, the operator should pay close attention to the area around the foramen ovale. Employing a large device in a small heart can increase the risk of arrhythmia such as atrial fibrillation as the device overlaps more of the atrial wall. Also, some closure devices can apply strain against the tissue and, with time, result in erosion. The most common location of erosion is anteriorly in the retro-aortic rim for an ASD device and aortic root. Uncommonly, a large, stiff device opposing the aorta can erode into the aortic root at the sinus of Valsalva with catastrophic outcomes. Finally, device fracture and wire perforations with hemopericardium have been reported, although rare.[22]

Unlike with ASD closure, pulmonary hypertension is not a common consideration when closing a PFO. However, in situations where the right atrial pressure is elevated, the operator can assess the effect of closing the PFO by inflating a low-pressure sizing balloon across the PFO until flow around the balloon is stopped. If the right atrial pressure rises significantly (>10 mm Hg), then the PFO is acting as a pop-off valve and should not be closed for concern of developing right heart failure.

UNUSUAL ANATOMIC CONSIDERATIONS

In situations where there are limitations to catheter access such as an occluded IVC or IVC filter, additional planning will be necessary based on the variation in anatomy. An IVC filter may present a challenge in passing a catheter from the femoral vein. If the filter could not be removed prior to the procedure, the authors recommend vascular ultrasound imaging of the femoral vein to ensure it is patent. Following that, injecting contrast into the femoral vein sheath can be performed to show flow through the IVC filter. To prevent trauma from recrossing the IVC filter, a long sheath through the IVC filter can be used prior to crossing the septum. The dilator is removed and adequate blood pull-back is done prior to advancing the wire across the septum and attempting to close the PFO. If there is concern about limiting the number of devices across the filter, TEE may be used instead of ICE.

While uncommon, closure of the PFO from the SVC is also possible. Due to the shape and direction of the PFO tunnel as described earlier, an SVC approach from the internal jugular vein poses some challenges in crossing both with the wire and with the closure device. Unlike the approach from the IVC, the guidewire does not have a direct path toward the septum, rather, as the SVC is directed caudal and anteriorly, a guidewire entering from the SVC is more likely to cross the tricuspid valve. An approach is to use a torquable catheter to retroflex the guidewire toward the PFO

tunnel. The wire then will take the usual route to cross the septum. Once the initial wire is across, the torquable catheter is exchanged for a more flexible catheter such as an MP1. The guidewire is then exchanged for a stiffer wire, such as an Amplatz extra-stiff wire. Withdrawing the torquable catheter must be done carefully so as not to displace the wire. Due to the upward pointing PFO tunnel, the wire will be under strain. The PFO can be modified using a sizing balloon to open the tunnel and make it easier to pass the closure device. Due to the direction of the SVC with respect to the septum, even with a modified PFO, there will be significant strain on the device as it exits the delivery sheath so imaging of both sides of the septum and ensuring that the septum primum and septum secundum are captured is important.

SUMMARY

A thorough understanding of the interatrial septal anatomy along with its assessment by different imaging modalities is critical in performing safe transcatheter PFO closure. PFO closures should be a low-risk procedure and is facilitated with TEE or ICE guidance, although there are operators who only use fluoroscopy with the Amplatzer device. The authors suggest performing a TEE prior to closure procedures to better appreciate the septal anatomy and to anticipate and rule out variables such as a small PFO or a long tunnel PFO, sinus venous ASD, pulmonary arterial-venous malformations, or unusual septal structures. This is complemented with intraoperative imaging, including a full ICE interrogation of the interatrial septum and agitated saline contrast study at the beginning of the procedure.

CLINICS CARE POINTS

- PFO is a common finding in the general population but may lead to serious conditions such as stroke from paradoxic embolism and platypnea orthodeoxia.

- Understanding the septal anatomy and position of the atrial septum in relation to the patient's long axis is vital for the safe closure of a PFO.

- Crossing the PFO is much more direct from the IVC as compared to the SVC due to the position of the atrial septum and the orientations of the IVC and SVC. Likewise crossing the PFO and performing a closure are much more direct from the IVC.

- Investigating the anatomy and right heart to left heart flows using TEE or ICE imaging must be done before undertaking closure of a PFO. This avoids missing pathology such as septum secundum ASD, pulmonary AVMs, or other causes for shunting.

DISCLOSURES

No funding sources for any of the authors. No commercial or financial conflicts of interest related to this article for Dr A. Mohammad and Dr H. Truong. Dr I. Abudayyeh is education faculty, Johnson and Johnson ICE.

REFERENCES

1. Hara H, Virmani R, Ladich E, et al. Patent foramen ovale: current pathology, pathophysiology, and clinical status. J Am Coll Cardiol 2005;46:1768–76.
2. Anderson RH, Brown NA, Webb S. Development and structure of the atrial septum. Heart 2002;88:104–10.
3. Koutroulou I, Tsivgoulis G, Tsalikakis D, et al. Epidemiology of patent foramen ovale in general population and in stroke patients: a narrative review. Front Neurol 2020;11:281.
4. Hanaoka T, Suyama K, Taguchi A, et al. Shifting of puncture site in the fossa ovalis during radiofrequency catheter ablation: intracardiac echocardiography-guided transseptal left heart catheterization. Jpn Heart J 2003;44:673–80.
5. Bidart C, Vaseghi M, Cesario DA, et al. Radiofrequency current delivery via transseptal needle to facilitate septal puncture. Heart Rhythm 2007;4:1573–6.
6. Calvert PA, Rana BS, Kydd AC, et al. Patent foramen ovale: anatomy, outcomes, and closure. Nat Rev Cardiol 2011;8:148–60.
7. Hagen PT, Scholz DG, Edwards WD. Incidence and size of patent foramen ovale during the first 10 decades of life: an autopsy study of 965 normal hearts. Mayo Clin Proc 1984;59:17–20.
8. McKenzie JA, Edwards WD, Hagler DJ. Anatomy of the patent foramen ovale for the interventionalist. Cathet Cardiovasc Interv 2009;73:821–6.
9. Ho SY, McCarthy KP, Rigby ML. Morphological features pertinent to interventional closure of patent oval foramen. J Intervent Cardiol 2003;16:33–8.
10. Rana BS, Shapiro LM, McCarthy KP, et al. Three-dimensional imaging of the atrial septum and patent foramen ovale anatomy: defining the morphological phenotypes of patent foramen ovale. Eur J Echocardiogr 2010;11:i19–25.
11. Yetkin E, Atalay H, Ileri M. Atrial septal aneurysm: prevalence and covariates in adults. Int J Cardiol 2016;223:656–9.
12. Snijder RJR, Luermans JGLM, de Heij AH, et al. Patent foramen ovale with atrial septal aneurysm is strongly associated with migraine with aura: a large observational study. J Am Heart Assoc 2016;5:e003771.
13. Turc G, Lee J-Y, Brochet E, et al. Atrial septal aneurysm, shunt size, and recurrent stroke risk in patients with patent foramen ovale. J Am Coll Cardiol 2020;75:2312–20.
14. Lefebvre B, Naidu S, Nathan AS, et al. Impact of echocardiographic parameters on recurrent stroke in the randomized REDUCE PFO cryptogenic stroke trial. Structural Heart 2021;5:367–75.
15. Hijazi ZM, Shivkumar K, Sahn DJ. Intracardiac echocardiography during interventional and electrophysiological cardiac catheterization. Circulation 2009;119:587–96.
16. Anon. Patent Foramen ovale closure for stroke, myocardial infarction, peripheral embolism, migraine, and hypoxemia. Elsevier; 2020.
17. Słodowska K, Hołda J, Dudkiewicz D, et al. Thickness of the left atrial wall surrounding the left atrial appendage orifice. J Cardiovasc Electrophysiol 2021;32:2262–8.
18. Schwinger ME, Gindea AJ, Freedberg RS, et al. The anatomy of the interatrial septum: a transesophageal echocardiographic study. Am Heart J 1990;119:1401–5.
19. Ren P, Xie M. Diagnostic accuracy of trans-thoracic echocardiography for patent foramen ovale: a systematic review and meta-analysis. Heart 2012;98:E304.
20. Mojadidi MK, Bogush N, Caceres JD, et al. Diagnostic accuracy of transesophageal echocardiogram for the detection of patent foramen ovale: a meta-analysis. Echocardiography 2014;31(6):752–8.
21. Mojadidi MK, Winoker JS, Roberts SC, et al. Accuracy of conventional transthoracic echocardiography for the diagnosis of intracardiac right-to-left shunt: a meta-analysis of prospective studies. Echocardiography 2014;31(9):1036–48.
22. Kumar P, Orford JL, Tobis JM. Two cases of pericardial tamponade due to nitinol wire fracture of a gore septal occluder. Cathet Cardiovasc Interv 2020;96:219–24.

Techniques for Identifying a Patent Foramen Ovale

Transthoracic Echocardiography, Transesophageal Echocardiography, Transcranial Doppler, Right Heart Catheterization

Sanaullah Mojaddedi, MD[a,b,1], Muhammad O. Zaman, MD[c],
Islam Y. Elgendy, MD[d], Mohammad K. Mojadidi, MD[e,*]

KEYWORDS

- Patent foramen ovale • PFO • Congenital heart defect • Right-to-left shunt
- Interventional cardiology • Echocardiography • Cardiovascular imaging

KEY POINTS

- Initial patent foramen ovale (PFO) diagnosis can be made using transthoracic echocardiography or transcranial Doppler (TCD) bubble study due to their noninvasive nature, safety, low cost, and high sensitivity (with TCD).
- Transesophageal echocardiography (TEE) bubble study is usually needed to confirm a PFO and assess the atrial septal anatomy, prior to PFO closure.
- Although TEE is considered by many as the reference standard for PFO diagnosis, it can miss or misdiagnose a PFO in 10% of cases; right heart catheterization can be utilized in selective cases where there is high clinical suspicion for a PFO but nondiagnostic noninvasive testing.

INTRODUCTION

The transition from fetal to adult circulation causes functional closure of the foramen ovale at birth, with complete atrial septal closure typically occurring by 7 months. However, in 20% to 25% of the population, the foramen ovale remains patent.[1,2] Transient intracardiac right-to-left shunting (RLS), across a patent foramen ovale (PFO), typically occurs during maneuvers that increase right atrium (RA) pressure, such as coughing or the Valsalva maneuver. Once considered clinically benign, PFO has been linked to various debilitating conditions, such as stroke in healthy young adults, peripheral embolism, migraine with aura, hypoxemia, and decompression sickness.[1,3,4]

With emerging clinical trials on therapeutic benefits of PFO closure to treat associated medical

Funding statement: This correspondence received no specific grant from any funding agency in the public, commercial, or not-for-profit sectors.

[a] University of Central Florida College of Medicine, Graduate Medical Education, Orlando, FL, USA; [b] Internal Medicine Residency Program, HCA Florida North Florida Hospital, 6500 West Newberry Road, Gainesville, FL 32605, USA; [c] Department of Cardiovascular Medicine, University of Louisville, University of Louisville Heart Hospital, 201 Abraham Flexner Way, Suite 600, Louisville, KY 40202, USA; [d] Division of Cardiovascular Medicine, Gill Heart Institute, University of Kentucky, UK Gill Heart & Vascular Institute, 800 Rose Street, First Floor, Suite G100, Lexington, KY 40536, USA; [e] Division of Cardiology, Department of Medicine, Virginia Commonwealth University (VCU Health), 1250 East Marshall Street, Richmond, VA 23219, USA

[1] Present address: 1147 Northwest 64th Terrace, Gainesville, FL 32605.

* Corresponding author.
E-mail address: mkmojadidi@gmail.com

Cardiol Clin 42 (2024) 473–486
https://doi.org/10.1016/j.ccl.2024.01.005
0733-8651/24/Published by Elsevier Inc.

conditions, particularly ischemic stroke related to PFO, there is a need for reliable imaging modalities to visualize, quantify, diagnose, and, if indicated, guide closure of the PFO. A number of diagnostic modalities are available for PFO imaging, each with their strengths and limitations. Transthoracic echocardiography (TTE) is the most commonly used initial screening test due to its availability, safety, and direct visualization of the atria.[5,6] An acceptable alternative with enhanced sensitivity is transcranial Doppler (TCD), an indirect technique virtually excluding a RLS with a negative test, albeit less accurate for distinguishing between a PFO, atrial septal defect, and pulmonary shunt when compared with transesophageal echocardiography (TEE).[1,4] TEE is largely considered the reference standard for PFO imaging, due to its superior image quality and close proximity of the ultrasound probe to the heart.[7,8] Unfortunately, TEE has a 10% false negative rate, likely due to the patients' inability to perform an adequate Valsalva maneuver when a probe is passed through the oropharynx. These imaging modalities utilize a bubble study, where agitated saline contrast is injected intravenously to demonstrate passage of bubbles across a PFO, from the RA to the left atrium (LA).[6,9] Cardiac computed tomography (CT) and cardiac MRI (CMR) are less common diagnostic approaches, given their inferior sensitivity compared with ultrasound-based imaging.[10] Intracardiac echocardiography (ICE), catheter probing, and angiography are invasive techniques that can complement the noninvasive modalities on a case-by-case basis, and guide percutaneous PFO closure.[5] This review article discusses the imaging modalities for detecting and quantifying a PFO, with emphasis on their advantages and limitations.

ULTRASONOGRAPHY

Evaluation of a PFO utilizing ultrasonography can be achieved with TTE, TEE, TCD, or ICE.[1,11] Utilization of an agitated saline bubble study with a provocation maneuver (ie, Valsalva, sniff, or cough) is necessary to reverse the interatrial pressure gradient, and demonstrate a PFO and the degree of shunting.[1,12] These imaging modalities can detect interatrial shunting either at the level of the atria (TTE, TEE, ICE) or embolic signals at the level of the middle cerebral arteries by TCD.[8,13] Large PFOs are readily visualized with color flow Doppler due to obvious left-to-right interatrial shunting without provocation maneuvers.[5,6]

CONTRAST AGENT FOR BUBBLE STUDY

During echocardiography, the ultrasonographer acquires an optimal view of the interatrial septum while an assistant prepares the contrast agent.[6,8] The most common contrast is saline that is agitated between two 10 cc syringes several times to create micro-air bubbles before injection. Adding 1 to 2 mL of the patient's blood in the agitated saline mixture can increase the study's sensitivity without compromising specificity.[14,15] The addition of blood introduces plasma proteins that coat the air bubbles and creates a foam, stabilizing the microbubbles and decreasing the negligible risk of air embolism from larger air bubbles.[9,16] Repeated contrast injections may be utilized for improved sensitivity.[17,18] Several other contrasts have been developed, yet agitated saline remains the most commonly used agent due to its availability, low cost, and ease of access.[9]

CHOOSING AN INJECTION SITE FOR BUBBLE STUDY (BRACHIAL OR FEMORAL)

The brachial vein in the arm has traditionally been used as the contrast injection site for PFO detection.[19] However, studies have shown that femoral vein injection has a higher sensitivity for PFO detection compared to brachial vein injection.[20] This is related to the direction of venous blood inflow into the RA. Contrast injection through the brachial vein enters the RA through the superior vena cava and directly crosses the tricuspid valve. In comparison, injection via the femoral vein enters the RA through the inferior vena cava and is directed to the superior aspect of the atrial septum, especially if a Eustachian valve is present, increasing the probability of trans-septal passage in case of a PFO.[21,22] Nonetheless, obtaining femoral vein access solely for agitated saline injection is usually impractical and carries an additional risk of line-associated infections compared to antecubital venous access.[5] Femoral vein access might be considered for patients with a high suspicion of PFO with negative imaging studies, especially in the presence of a Eustachian valve in the RA.[6] Thus, the brachial vein remains more practical for most patients without femoral venous access. In the cardiac catheterization laboratory, a femoral vein injection becomes practical and is preferable for assessing the degree of flow across the PFO. We usually decrease the amount of air in the syringe to less than 0.5 mL when injecting from the femoral vein because the amount of air crossing the septum becomes appreciable.

PROVOCATION MANEUVERS DURING A BUBBLE STUDY

At rest, the left atrial pressure is higher than the RA pressure. A Valsalva maneuver is performed to

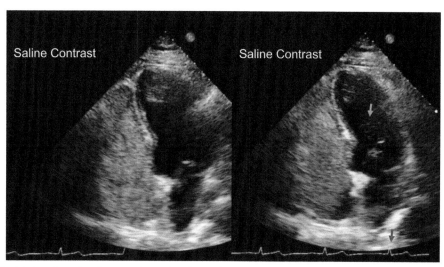

Fig. 1. Apical 4 chamber view by transthoracic echocardiogram, illustrating a positive bubble study. In the image on the left, the agitated saline bubbles are seen in the right atrium and right ventricle. In the image on the right, saline contrast (*blue arrow*) is visualized in the left ventricle before the third cardiac cycle (*red arrow*), indicative of an intracardiac right-to-left shunt (PFO or atrial septal defect). Microbubbles opacifying the right ventricle and the right atrium with passage of less than 10 microbubbles within 1 cardiac cycle. (Adapted with permission from Gad et al., Echocardiography, Transcranial Doppler, and Oximetry for Imaging and Quantification of PFO-Mediated Shunts, Mojadidi et al, Patent Foramen Ovale Closure for Stroke, Myocardial Infarction, Peripheral Embolism, Migraine, and Hypoxemia, 15-28, London, Elsevier, 2020.)

transiently alter the interatrial pressure and thus demonstrate a RLS. After immediate release of the Valsalva maneuver, the pressure gradient reverses with increased venous return, resulting in an elevated RA pressure. This enables blood to flow through the PFO, and the transient RLS can be visualized as it crosses from the RA to LA.[23] For unconscious or semiunconscious patients, performing the Valsalva maneuver may be difficult. Therefore, gentle right upper quadrant pressure may be applied for 15 to 20 seconds, with release upon contrast injection and RA opacification.[24,25] A provocation maneuver should always be utilized to increase the sensitivity of diagnostic echocardiography.[26,27]

DIAGNOSTIC CRITERIA FOR INTRACARDIAC RIGHT-TO-LEFT SHUNT

The diagnostic process involves detecting microbubbles traversing the interatrial septum from the venous to the systemic circulation (**Fig. 1**). This RLS is directly visualized at the atrial level using TTE, TEE, and ICE, whereas TCD will detect embolic systemic microbubbles at the level of the middle cerebral arteries. If an adequate insonation window cannot be obtained during TCD, the carotid artery or any artery in the body will demonstrate the shunt, albeit unable to quantitate the degree of shunting. Although the exact number of microbubbles necessary for diagnosing a PFO

is not clearly established, most studies consider the presence of 1 or more microbubbles in the LA within 3 to 5 cardiac cycles following contrast medium injection and provocation confirms the presence of a RLS (see **Fig. 1**).[7,8] The echocardiographic literature perpetuates the misconception that the presence of microbubbles in the LA after 3 cardiac cycles suggests the existence of an intrapulmonary shunt.[8,13] But interventional cardiologists see this late crossing of bubbles frequently in the presence of a PFO documented during a right heart catheterization, as a PFO may open any time during the bubble study.[5] In 1500 TCD studies performed at the University of California, Los Angeles, the confirmed diagnosis of a pulmonary arteriovenous malformation occurred in only 1% of cases, the other 99% of positive studies were due to a PFO.[28] Although a positive TCD is not specific for a PFO, it is more likely that a positive TCD indicates the presence of a PFO. The incidence of an undiagnosed atrial septal defect (ASD) in adults is rare. The only proviso is in patients with hereditary hemorrhagic telangiectasia where the prevalence of pulmonary arteriovenous malformation is 30%.[28] The international consensus criteria for RLS may be used to grade the severity of the shunt (**Table 1**).[1,29] The specific criteria for a positive TCD diagnosis are discussed later. Of note, most studies that have established these criteria have not confirmed a

Table 1 The international consensus for grading right-to-left shunt severity with echocardiography	
Grade	**Microbubbles**
0	None
1	1–10
2	10–20
3	>20–snowstorm appearance of microbubbles

PFO using right heart catheterization, which leads to some false-positive and false-negative bubble studies.[5]

There will be a guidelines committee of the American Society of Echocardiography, the Society of Cardiac Angiography and Interventions, and the American Association of Neurology to reevaluate these issues and provide guidance for echocardiographic contrast studies interpretation. Major concerns for the committee include the timing of agitated saline bubbles in the LA that is inaccurate for distinguishing a PFO from a pulmonary arteriovenous malformation, inaccurate sizing of a PFO with TTE and TEE compared to right heart catheterization, and discussion regarding right heart catheterization becoming the true gold standard for PFO diagnosis due to significant false-negative and false-positive studies with all modes of echocardiography.

TRANSTHORACIC ECHOCARDIOGRAPHY FOR THE DIAGNOSIS OF PATENT FORAMEN OVALE

TTE is the primary imaging modality employed for PFO screening due to its widespread availability and low cost.[1,6,27]

Protocol for a Transthoracic Echocardiographic Bubble Study

1. The echocardiography probe is placed at the apical 4 chamber or subcostal view, and an optimal view is obtained.
2. Agitated saline or a contrast agent is injected via the antecubital vein (or femoral access if available), followed by prolonged TTE image acquisition.
3. The study is repeated with a provocation maneuver, such as Valsalva. A positive test is indicated when microbubbles traverse the atrial septum or are observed in the LA/ventricle within 1 to 5 cardiac cycles, following complete opacification of the RA.

Diagnostic Accuracy of Transthoracic Echocardiography Bubble Study

The sensitivity and specificity of the TTE bubble study are affected by several factors pertaining to the imaging modality itself and the protocol utilized. According to a meta-analysis including 13 prospective studies (1436 patients), TTE with fundamental B-mode imaging has a weighted sensitivity of 46.4% (95% confidence interval [CI], 41.1%–51.8%) with a specificity of 99.2% (95% CI, 98.4%–99.7%) when compared with TEE for detecting a RLS.[30] The outcomes remained consistent across various contrast agents, with different cutoffs for defining a positive test based on minimum microbubbles, and different cutoffs for determining a positive study based on the number of cardiac cycles.[30]

Modern echocardiography is generally performed with harmonic imaging, allowing better-quality images. A meta-analysis of 15 prospective studies (1995 patients) revealed that TTE with harmonic imaging demonstrated a sensitivity of 90.5% (95% CI, 88.1%–92.6%) and specificity of 92.6% (95% CI, 91.0%–94.0%) when compared to TEE as the reference.[1,31] The inclusion of a small quantity of the patients' blood in the agitated saline mixture enhanced sensitivity without affecting specificity. Furthermore, a cutoff of 1 or more microbubbles (in comparison to ≥5) within 3 cardiac cycles (in comparison to 5) improved the specificity of TTE with harmonic imaging without compromising sensitivity[1,31] (**Table 2**). When interpreting these data, it is important to note that any study that utilizes TEE bubble study as the reference for PFO diagnosis is fundamentally flawed, since the accurate comparator is right heart catheterization with the passage of a guidewire, catheter, or iodinated contrast through the PFO.[5] Only a few studies have used right heart catheterization as the gold standard. Therefore, TEE commonly is used as the comparator in most studies due to its partially invasive nature and superior visualization of the atrial septal anatomy, offering added anatomic information regarding the PFO when compared with TTE.

Advantages and Limitations of Transthoracic Echocardiography for Detecting a Patent Foramen Ovale

A TTE bubble study offers advantages such as high specificity, noninvasive nature, easy availability, and low cost (compared to TEE), making it the first choice in most centers for PFO screening. Limitations of TTE include inadequate acoustic windows, limited resolution, and challenges in visualizing the interatrial septum (**Table 3**).

Table 2
Diagnostic accuracies of transthoracic echocardiography (with and without harmonic imaging), transcranial Doppler, and transesophageal echocardiography bubble studies for the detection of intracardiac right-to-left shunt*

Imaging Modality	Sensitivity	Specificity	LR$^+$	LR$^-$
TTE-F	46	99	20.85	0.57
TTE-HI	91	93	13.52	0.13
TCD	97	93	13.51	0.04
TEE	89	91	5.92	0.22

*TTE-F, transthoracic echocardiography with fundamental imaging; TTE-HI, transthoracic echocardiography with harmonic imaging; LR+, positive likelihood ratio; LR, negative likelihood ratio.

TTE-F, TTE-HI, and TCD compared with TEE as the reference standard. TEE compared with PFO confirmation by cardiac catheterization, surgery, and/or autopsy as the reference standard.

Adapted with permission from Gad et al., Echocardiography, Transcranial Doppler, and Oximetry for Imaging and Quantification of PFO-Mediated Shunts, Mojadidi et al, Patent Foramen Ovale Closure for Stroke, Myocardial Infarction, Peripheral Embolism, Migraine, and Hypoxemia, 15-28, London, Elsevier, 2020.

Clinicians should not rely on a TTE alone, as a PFO may be missed. Instead, a combination of TTE or TCD should be utilized for screening, followed by a TEE for confirmation.[32,33]

TRANSESOPHAGEAL ECHOCARDIOGRAPHY FOR THE DIAGNOSIS OF PATENT FORAMEN OVALE

Many clinicians consider TEE the reference standard for diagnosing and quantifying RLS mediated by a PFO. TEE enables direct visualization of the atrial septal anatomy, facilitating the identification of an atrial septal aneurysm, the presence of a Eustachian valve or a Chiari network (**Fig. 2**), and the assessment of shunt severity.[34,35] A PFO accompanied by an atrial septal aneurysm or a large shunt has been associated with an increased risk of stroke.[36,37] Furthermore, TEE can differentiate between a PFO and an ASD, although it may still have limitations in diagnosing pulmonary shunts accurately. TEE offers the additional advantage of detecting other potential sources of embolism, such as left atrial appendage thrombus, left ventricular thrombus, or atherosclerotic aortic plaque, which are often overlooked by TTE.[35,38]

Protocol for a Transesophageal Echocardiographic Bubble Study

1. To enhance patient comfort, topical pharyngeal anesthesia can be administered 15 minutes before TEE probe insertion. After esophageal intubation, the interatrial septum is visualized in multiple projections using multiplane angles. Bicaval, 4 chamber, short and long axis views accurately assess the interatrial septum anatomy.
2. The short axis and bicaval views offer direct visualization of the PFO (**Fig. 3**A).
3. As with TTE, agitated saline or a contrast agent is injected intravenously. Performing a Valsalva maneuver may be difficult for semiconscious or sedated patients with a probe in their esophagus. Moderate right upper quadrant abdominal pressure can be applied for 10 to 20 seconds, followed by pressure release immediately after RA opacification with microbubbles, to increase venous return and RA pressure.
4. A positive test is defined by at least one microbubble in the LA with a momentary opening of the PFO flap during the first 3 cardiac cycles following contrast agent injection and complete right atrial opacification. Documentation of bubbles (see **Fig. 1**) or color Doppler flow (**Fig. 3**B) across the PFO canal is pathognomonic. The international consensus for echocardiographic grading (see **Table 1**) is used to quantify the size of the shunts for both TTE and TEE bubble studies.

Diagnostic Accuracy of Transesophageal Echocardiography Bubble Study

According to one observational study that compared TEE with confirmation of PFO by autopsy, TEE demonstrated a sensitivity of 89%.[39] A meta-analysis comparing TEE to PFO confirmed by surgery, right heart catheterization, and/or autopsy found that TEE had a weighted sensitivity of 89% and specificity of 91%.[40] Even though TEE is considered the reference standard, relying solely on TEE may result in missed or misdiagnosis of PFO in approximately 10% of cases.

Advantages and Limitations of Transesophageal Echocardiography for Detecting a Patent Foramen Ovale

The utilization of TEE for diagnosing a PFO offers several benefits, including direct visualization of the atrial septal anatomy, differentiation between a ASD and PFO, detection of a Eustachian valve or Chiari network (see **Fig. 2**), identification of an

Table 3
Advantages and limitations of transthoracic echocardiography, transcranial Doppler, transesophageal echocardiography, intracardiac echocardiography, and angiography for the diagnosis of PFO

Imaging Modality	Advantages	Limitations
TTE	• Readily available • Cost-effective • Excellent safety • Easy to perform	• Low resolution • Less sensitive than TCD • Images may be limited by patient's body habitus and poor echocardiographic windows • Often difficult to differentiate between PFO, ASD, and pulmonary shunts
TCD	• Highly sensitive • Cost-effective • Excellent safety • Easy to perform	• Positive test based on an arbitrary cutoff • Inability to differentiate between PFO, ASD, and pulmonary shunts (ie, lower specificity) • Inability to visualize atrial septum
TEE	• Highly accurate imaging modality • Can visualize atrial septal anatomy • Accurate assessment of PFO size • Accurate assessment of shunt severity • Differentiates PFO from ASD and pulmonary shunts • Useful for closure planning • In addition to diagnosing PFO, can detect other sources of embolism	• Semi-invasive procedure • Need for sedation • Difficulty performing Valsalva with a probe in the esophagus while typically being sedated • Carries a risk of complications • May not be used in patients with esophageal stricture, diverticula, cancer, or varices • Difficulty in uncooperative patients with swallowing dysfunction
ICE	• Detailed visualization of atrial septal anatomy • Allows guidance during device deployment • Residual shunt assessment post-PFO closure • Performance without general anesthesia • Second operator not needed	• Need for second venous access • Increased risk of vascular access-related complications • Possible limitations by operator inexperience

Adapted with permission from Gad et al., Echocardiography, Transcranial Doppler, and Oximetry for Imaging and Quantification of PFO-Mediated Shunts, Mojadidi et al, Patent Foramen Ovale Closure for Stroke, Myocardial Infarction, Peripheral Embolism, Migraine, and Hypoxemia, 15-28, London, Elsevier, 2020.

atrial septal aneurysm, measurement of PFO size, and evaluation of shunt severity with bubble study or color flow Doppler. However, sedation may increase procedural risk, particularly in patients with impaired left ventricular function. Additionally, TEE carries a small risk of esophagus-related complications such as perforation and bleeding, especially in patients with pre-existing esophageal conditions (strictures, diverticula, cancer, varices, and achalasia).[41] A summary of the advantages and limitations of TEE in PFO detection is provided in **Table 3**.

TEE demonstrates acceptable diagnostic accuracy compared to autopsy, right heart catheterization, and PFO detection during surgery. Its superiority lies in providing detailed anatomic information about the PFO and excluding non-PFO-mediated RLS. After an initial noninvasive screening for RLS, using TTE or TCD, TEE serves as a good confirmatory test for detecting and quantifying PFO-mediated shunting. However, it is essential to recognize that relying exclusively on TEE for PFO diagnosis may be misleading if only a few bubbles are observed in the LA. A right

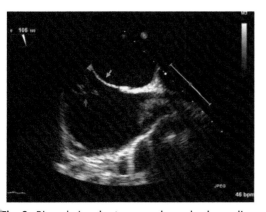

Fig. 2. Bicaval view by transesophageal echocardiography showing an atrial septum that proved aneurysmal during motion (*blue arrow*) with the presence of a Chiari network (*red arrow*). (Adapted with permission from Gad et al., Echocardiography, Transcranial Doppler, and Oximetry for Imaging and Quantification of PFO-Mediated Shunts, Mojadidi et al, Patent Foramen Ovale Closure for Stroke, Myocardial Infarction, Peripheral Embolism, Migraine, and Hypoxemia, 15-28, London, Elsevier, 2020.)

heart catheterization may be necessary for a correct diagnosis based on clinical indications.[42,43]

TRANSCRANIAL DOPPLER FOR THE DIAGNOSIS OF PATENT FORAMEN OVALE

Whereas TTE and TEE provide direct visualization of the atrial septum, a TCD bubble study allows for indirect screening of a PFO by detecting a RLS. Like TTE, administering an intravenous contrast agent, such as agitated saline, combined with a Valsalva maneuver, allows for identifying a RLS. With TCD, insonation of the middle cerebral arteries following contrast injection and a Valsalva measured with a manometer allow functional assessment of the RLS (**Fig. 4**). The degree of shunting may be classified with the Spencer logarithmic scale, where the severity is scored from 0 to 5, with 0 indicating no shunt and 5 indicating a large shunt (**Table 4**). Score grades 3 to 5 are considered positive for clinically significant PFO with a TCD bubble study, as these correspond to the presence of a PFO during right heart catheterization. Grades 1 to 2 usually indicate clinically insignificant pulmonary shunts or pinhole septal defects[29,44] (**Fig. 5**).

Protocol for a Transcranial Doppler Bubble Study

1. The TCD ultrasound probe is placed through an identified acoustic window (ie, transtemporal, transorbital, or suboccipital).
2. The patient performs a Valsalva maneuver while an agitated saline mixture is intravenously injected. This is done with the subject exhaling forcefully into a tube connected to a manometer, maintaining a pressure of 40 mm Hg for 10 seconds. Adding 1 mL of the patient's blood

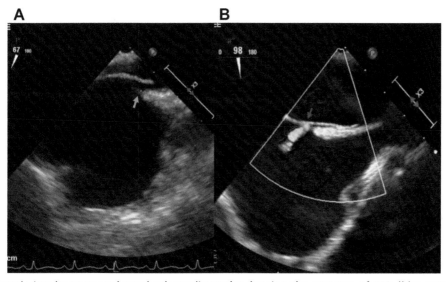

Fig. 3. Bicaval view by transesophageal echocardiography showing the presence of PFO (*blue arrow*) that is partially open (*A*) resulting in baseline left-to-right shunting, indicated by the Doppler color flow across the PFO (*red arrow*) (*B*). (Adapted with permission from Gad et al., Echocardiography, Transcranial Doppler, and Oximetry for Imaging and Quantification of PFO-Mediated Shunts, Mojadidi et al, Patent Foramen Ovale Closure for Stroke, Myocardial Infarction, Peripheral Embolism, Migraine, and Hypoxemia, 15-28, London, Elsevier, 2020.)

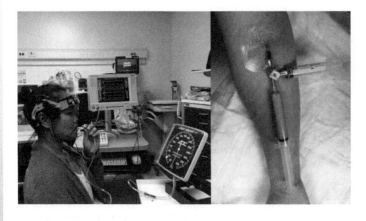

Fig. 4. Left: A patient is seen wearing a transcranial Doppler headset that has bilateral ultrasound probes mounted at the level of the temples, for insonation of the middle cerebral arteries. The patient is seen performing a Valsalva maneuver using visual feedback with the aid of a manometer. Right: A 3 way stopcock is used to prepare the agitated saline–blood mixture, which is intravenously injected immediately before release of the Valsalva maneuver. (Adapted with permission from Gad et al., Echocardiography, Transcranial Doppler, and Oximetry for Imaging and Quantification of PFO-Mediated Shunts, Mojadidi et al, Patent Foramen Ovale Closure for Stroke, Myocardial Infarction, Peripheral Embolism, Migraine, and Hypoxemia, 15-28, London, Elsevier, 2020.)

or a dedicated echocardiographic contrast medium can enhance the study's sensitivity.

3. If a RLS is present, the circulating microbubbles in the insonated artery can be visualized using M-mode Doppler. The shunt is quantified over 1 minute using the Spencer scale.

4. Although this method is not validated, a carotid artery can be used for insonation if the cerebral arteries cannot be identified. The carotid artery can demonstrate a RLS, but it cannot be used to quantify the degree of shunt.

Diagnostic Accuracy of Transcranial Doppler Bubble Study

TCD bubble study is a very sensitive modality for detecting RLS. Some studies reported a higher sensitivity with TCD than TEE, when PFO confirmation with a right heart catheterization (PFO probing with a guidewire under fluoroscopy) was used as the reference.[29,44] One large meta-analysis of 27 prospective studies (1968 patients) reported the TCD bubble study to have a sensitivity of 97% and a specificity of 93% for detecting

intracardiac RLS when compared with TEE as the reference.[45] Power M-mode software in modern TCD machines improves microbubble signal detection, enhancing the accuracy of right-to-left shunt quantification. In a study by Spencer and colleagues, power M-mode TCD demonstrated higher sensitivity and accuracy for detecting intracardiac right-to-left shunt than older TCD models without power M-mode compared to TEE.[44] A recent study analyzed a novel robotic TCD ultrasound device for RLS detection compared with conventional TCD, which demonstrated comparable accuracy without the need of a trained registered vascular technologist.[46] The diagnostic accuracy of TCD for detecting intracardiac RLS is summarized in **Table 2**.

Advantages and Limitations of Transcranial Echocardiography for Detecting a Patent Foramen Ovale

TCD is easily performed, highly sensitive, and affordable. These characteristics position TCD as an excellent initial screening test for PFO detection. Nevertheless, a positive TCD result, while indicative of a right-to-left shunt, may not necessarily confirm the presence of a PFO. False-positive outcomes can arise due to an ASD or pulmonary shunt. A pulmonary arteriovenous malformation is observed in 1% of positive TCD studies unless the investigation involves individuals with suspected hereditary hemorrhagic telangiectasia. Therefore, 99% of grade 3 or higher TCD bubble studies are due to the presence of an intracardiac RLS (PFO or ASD). Since TCD utilizes an indirect functional approach that does not directly visualize the atrial septum, a positive test typically necessitates a subsequent confirmatory assessment using

Table 4
The spencer logarithmic scale for transcranial Doppler grading

Grade	Microbubbles	Interpretation
0	0	No shunt
1	1–10	Insignificant shunt
2	11–30	Insignificant shunt
3	31–100	Positive shunt
4	101–300	Positive for shunt, moderate to large
5	<300	Positive for large shunt

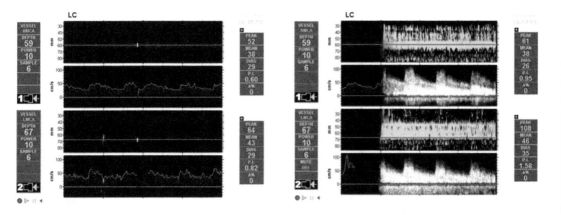

Grade 1 Rest   Grade 5 Valsalva

Fig. 5. Transcranial Doppler grading with microembolic signals that measure the degree of right-to-left shunting ranging from grade 1 (*left*) to grade 5 (*right*). (Adapted with permission from Gad et al., Echocardiography, Transcranial Doppler, and Oximetry for Imaging and Quantification of PFO-Mediated Shunts, Mojadidi et al, Patent Foramen Ovale Closure for Stroke, Myocardial Infarction, Peripheral Embolism, Migraine, and Hypoxemia, 15-28, London, Elsevier, 2020.)

TEE or ICE (during percutaneous PFO device closure). However, given its high sensitivity and negative predictive value, a negative TCD study virtually excludes an intracardiac shunt. TEE is unlikely to be diagnostic when a patient presents with a clinically suggestive history of PFO with a negative TCD bubble study. Depending on the strength of the clinical circumstances, a right heart catheterization may be warranted to investigate the possibility of a guidewire passing through the atrial septum into the LA, thus providing valuable diagnostic information. The advantages and disadvantages of TCD for intracardiac RLS detection are summarized in **Table 3**.

INTRACARDIAC ECHOCARDIOGRAPHY FOR THE DIAGNOSIS OF PATENT FORAMEN OVALE

ICE is an additional imaging modality used for direct anatomic visualization of the atrial septum and estimation of RLS severity.[47] Predominately utilized during percutaneous PFO closure, ICE provides practical guidance for occluder device placement and assessment of postclosure residual shunting. A horizontal view of the septum posterior to the aortic bulge enables clear visualization of a PFO. It is beneficial in assessing the inferior vena cava rim and the inferior aspect of the interatrial septum, which may pose challenges with TEE.[48] ICE has several advantages making it particularly useful during PFO closure; these include detailed direct visualization of the atrial septal anatomy, performance without general anesthesia, guidance during device deployment,

residual shunt assessment post-PFO closure, and the interventionalist's ability to control the ICE probe during the procedure without the need for another specialist. Disadvantages of ICE include increased procedural cost, the need for a second venous access, increased risk of vascular access-related complications, and possible limitations by operator inexperience.[49]

In a study by Van and colleagues, it was observed that the detection rate of preclosure RLS was comparable between ICE and TCD. However, following closure, ICE failed to identify 34% of small residual shunts detected by TCD.[50] This discrepancy can be attributed to the monoplane nature of ICE, or the reduced image yield caused by an occluder device obstructing the passage of contrast microbubbles.

Although ICE is not routinely utilized for PFO diagnosis, like TCD or TTE bubble studies, it offers a unique insight into the cardiac anatomy during PFO closure making it an acceptable imaging tool comparable to TEE. The clinician should assess whether ICE or TEE is best for the patient. Generally, for patients with contraindications to anesthesia and intubation, ICE is better suited. TEE would allow an increased temporal resolution with comprehensive cardiac visualization, but at the cost of sedation, intubation, and possible trauma to the gastrointestinal tract.[51]

EAR OXIMETRY FOR THE DIAGNOSIS OF PATENT FORAMEN OVALE

The indirect assessment of right-to-left shunt using ear oximetry was initially described by Lüthy and colleagues over 50 years ago, but its clinical validation remains incomplete. In their 1959 study, Lüthy and colleagues observed temporary arterial oxygen desaturation in the earlobe of individuals with various congenital heart defects, including those with a RLS.[52] Subsequent studies have also reported transient arterial desaturation measured by ear oximetry following the Valsalva maneuver in patients with a PFO. Karttunen and colleagues conducted a study to assess the accuracy of ear oximetry in detecting PFO when compared to TEE as the reference. Their analysis included 83 patients and revealed a sensitivity of 85% and specificity of 100% for the ear oximetry method.[53] However, it is essential to note that this study was limited to a small cohort of cryptogenic stroke patients with a high pretest probability for a PFO. Despite the advantages of being easily performed, safe, and cost-effective, more extensive observational studies have failed to replicate the high diagnostic accuracy of ear oximetry alone for PFO detection.[54]

A study by Devendra and colleagues discovered 34% of included patients experienced a drop in oxygen saturation to less than 90% following stress testing.[55] PFO closure resulted in oxygen saturation improvement by $10.1 \pm 4.2\%$ ($P<.001$) and New York Heart Association functional class improved by a median of 1.5 classes.[55] This study emphasizes that a large RLS through a PFO is a form of cyanotic congenital heart disease, which should justify closure in symptomatic patients even in the absence of a paradoxic embolic event.

Consequently, while the ear oximetry method shows promise, further research is required to establish its clinical utility and validate its diagnostic accuracy. At present, it should be regarded as a supplementary tool rather than a stand-alone method for PFO detection.

CARDIAC COMPUTED TOMOGRAPHY FOR THE DIAGNOSIS OF PATENT FORAMEN OVALE

Cardiac CT has witnessed an upsurge in its application for cardiac imaging in recent years, including its potential use for detecting PFO. Unlike echocardiographic imaging, which relies on provocation maneuvers to demonstrate RLS, cardiac CT can diagnose PFO by visualizing the contrast that appears in the LA during the resting state.[56,57] The diagnostic performance of cardiac CT for PFO detection has been evaluated in several studies. Kim and colleagues reported that compared to TEE as the reference, cardiac CT exhibited a low sensitivity of 73% and a specificity of 98%, limiting its utility as a primary

screening modality for PFO detection in routine clinical practice.[56] Another observational study comparing cardiac CT to TTE found that cardiac CT had a sensitivity of 53% and specificity of 75% for PFO detection. Despite these limitations, cardiac CT offered improved imaging of the interatrial septum and enhanced identification of other septal variations, such as atrial septal aneurysm.[57]

Consequently, cardiac CT is not considered a sufficient imaging modality for identifying or quantifying PFO-mediated RLS. While it provides valuable anatomic information and detailed visualization of the interatrial septum, its diagnostic accuracy falls short compared to TEE and TTE. Future research may refine its capabilities and establish its role in the evaluation of PFO.

MRI FOR THE DIAGNOSIS OF PATENT FORAMEN OVALE

In recent years, CMR has emerged as a valuable diagnostic tool for various cardiac conditions and is undergoing extensive evaluation for multiple applications. However, its role in detecting PFO remains limited due to its lower sensitivity than TEE. The decreased diagnostic yield of CMR for PFO detection can be attributed to the absence of continuous and prolonged imaging necessary for diagnosis, as provocation maneuvers are not feasible. This limitation is significant because PFO-mediated RLS typically occurs transiently during the cardiac cycle.[10] Although the Amplatzer PFO occluder (Abbott; Chicago, IL) and the Gore Cardioform device (W.L. Gore & Associates; Newark, DE) are nonferromagnetic and are not dangerous in an MRI machine, CMR is suboptimal for assessing residual shunts post-PFO closure due to imaging artifacts caused by the occluder devices.[58,59] These artifacts interfere with the accurate visualization and evaluation of residual shunts, diminishing the effectiveness of CMR for this purpose.

SUMMARY AND RECOMMENDATIONS

Among the imaging modalities discussed, TCD and TTE bubble studies offer the highest sensitivity for detecting a PFO-mediated RLS, making them practical screening tests. They are both versatile semi-invasive techniques with low cost. Modern TTE with harmonic imaging tends to be available at most institutions, especially with the rise in ultrasonography use; the literature reports a sensitivity of up to 90% for detecting a PFO, but it may not provide sufficient information in obese patients or those with poor echocardiographic windows. In our clinical practice, TTE sensitivity appeared closer to 50% to 60%. We saw a significant portion of our patients with PFO screened with TTE to be false-negative, with a subsequent positive TEE or balloon sizing at the time of right heart catheterization. The literature's overestimation of TTE's sensitivity may, in part, be explained by the use of TEE as the reference standard, which itself can miss or misdiagnose a PFO in 10% of cases.[40]

TCD has a high negative predictive value but cannot differentiate between PFO, ASD, or pulmonary shunt. Robotic TCD devices may make the technology more available without requiring a trained registered vascular technologist. It is clinically useful as an initial screening test for PFO detection and for assessing for post device closure RLS. TEE offers superior image quality and sensitivity, making it the reference standard for PFO diagnosis. Still, it is semi-invasive, uncomfortable for the patient, and may carry minor risks. Performing a TEE before PFO closure helps confirm the diagnosis and provides valuable information on the atrial septal anatomy and high-risk features. ICE can be utilized during percutaneous PFO closure for patients unable to undergo TEE providing real-time imaging. During right heart catheterization, using angiography or visualizing a guidewire crossing the atrial septum under fluoroscopy remains an accurate but invasive method to confirm a PFO. A right heart catheterization should be the method against which all echocardiographic studies be compared. It allows for immediate ad hoc device closure without prior imaging. Cardiac CT and CMR have limited use, given their low sensitivity and high cost compared to other imaging options.[60]

The stroke neurologists at UCLA prefer to screen for a PFO in young individuals (aged $\leq$ 60 years) with suspected paradoxic embolism using a TCD bubble study followed by confirmation with TEE. ICE imaging is useful for guidance of PFO closure procedures, and assessment of residual RLS post device closure. When noninvasive imaging with TCD, TTE, and TEE remains inconclusive, a right heart catheterization (septal probing with a guidewire) can be utilized for invasive confirmation of a PFO, in selective cases where there is high clinical suspicion for PFO-associated stroke. Coexisting conditions that should increase the suspicion that a stroke is PFO associated include young patients who have multifocal cerebral infarcts, stroke after straining, deep vein thrombosis, an atrial septal aneurysm, Eustachian valve or Chiari network, or migraine with aura. The presence of one or more of these factors especially raises the suspicion that a PFO is the underlying pathway of stroke. The guidelines committee of the American Society of Echocardiography, the Society of Cardiac Angiography and Interventions, and the American Association of Neurology will address the weaknesses of current guidelines for PFO diagnosis and closure with uniformly updated guidelines to assist clinicians in decision-making.

The accurate diagnosis of a PFO relies on various imaging modalities. TTE, TEE, TCD, and ICE each have their advantages and limitations. The choice of modality depends on the clinical context, patient characteristics, and the need for additional information. The use of contrast agents, provocation maneuvers, and diagnostic criteria, such as the presence of microbubbles, helps enhance the accuracy of PFO detection. Understanding the strengths and weaknesses of these imaging techniques is crucial for clinicians to make informed decisions and provide appropriate treatment for patients with PFO-related complications.

CLINICS CARE POINTS

- TTE bubble study is generally considered the optimal initial screening imaging modality for PFO diagnosis due to its ease of use, availability, acceptable sensitivity (approximately 50% in clinical practice), and ability to visualize the atria. It is also widely available.

- TCD bubble study offers the highest sensitivity among imaging modalities for PFO diagnosis but is unable to visualize the atria or differentiate between a PFO, ASD, or pulmonary shunt.

- TEE bubble study is considered the reference standard by echocardiographers for detecting a PFO and is typically performed following a screening test.

- Interventional cardiologists believe the true gold standard for PFO diagnosis is a right heart catheterization with the ability to pass a guidewire across the atrial septum under fluoroscopy.

- Using intravenous agitated saline contrast and performing a Valsalva maneuver during an imaging study increases sensitivity without compromising specificity.

- Right heart catheterization is an invasive modality to diagnose a PFO when clinical suspicion is high with inconclusive noninvasive imaging.

- PFO screening is crucial in the correct population, which is usually younger individuals less than 60 years of age with a history of unprovoked stroke.

DISCLOSURE

This research was supported in whole or in part by HCA Healthcare, United States and/or an HCA Healthcare affiliated entity. The views expressed in this publication represent those of the authors and do not necessarily represent the official views of HCA Healthcare or any of its affiliated entities.

REFERENCES

1. Liu F, Kong Q, Zhang X, et al. Comparative analysis of the diagnostic value of several methods for the diagnosis of patent foramen ovale. Echocardiography 2021;38(5):790-7.

2. Hagen PT, Scholz DG, Edwards WD. Incidence and size of patent foramen ovale during the first 10 decades of life: an autopsy study of 965 normal hearts. Mayo Clin Proc 1984;59(1):17-20.

3. Hara H, Virmani R, Ladich E, et al. Patent foramen ovale: current pathology, pathophysiology, and clinical status. J Am Coll Cardiol 2005;46(9):1768-76.

4. Arfaras-Melainis A, Palaiodimos L, Mojadidi MK. Transcatheter closure of patent foramen ovale. Interv Cardiol Clin 2019;8(4):341-56.

5. Available at:Patent foramen ovale closure for stroke, Myocardial infarction, peripheral embolism, migraine, and hypoxemia. Elsevier; 2020 https://linkinghub.elsevier.com/retrieve/pii/C20180020162. [Accessed 2 April 2023].

6. Van der Giessen H, Wilson LC, Coffey S, et al. Review: detection of patient foramen ovale using transcranial Doppler or standard echocardiography. Australas J Ultrasound Med 2020;23(4):210-9.

7. Teshome MK, Najib K, Nwagbara CC, et al. Patent foramen ovale: a comprehensive review. Curr Probl Cardiol 2020;45(2):100392.

8. Miranda B, Fonseca AC, Ferro JM. Patent foramen ovale and stroke. J Neurol 2018;265(8):1943-9.

9. Zhao E, Cheng G, Zhang Y, et al. Comparison of different contrast agents in detecting cardiac right-to-left shunt in patients with a patent foramen ovale during contrast-transthoracic echocardiography. BioMed Res Int 2017;2017:6086094.

10. Hamilton-Craig C, Sestito A, Natale L, et al. Contrast transoesophageal echocardiography remains superior to contrast-enhanced cardiac magnetic resonance imaging for the diagnosis of patent foramen ovale. Eur J Echocardiogr 2011;12(3):222-7.

11. Borowy CS, Mukhdomi T. Sonography Physical Principles and Instrumentation. In: StatPearls. StatPearls Publishing; 2023. http://www.ncbi.nlm.nih.gov/books/NBK567710/. [Accessed 13 April 2023].

12. Collado FMS, Poulin M, Murphy JJ, et al. Patent foramen ovale closure for stroke prevention and other Disorders. J Am Heart Assoc 2018;7(12):e007146.

13. Mahmoud AN, Elgendy IY, Agarwal N, et al. Identification and Quantification of patent foramen ovale–mediated shunts. Interv Cardiol Clin 2017;6(4):495-504.

14. Fan S, Nagai T, Luo H, et al. Superiority of the combination of blood and agitated saline for routine contrast enhancement. J Am Soc Echocardiogr Off Publ Am Soc Echocardiogr 1999;12(2):94-8.

15. Jeon DS, Luo H, Iwami T, et al. The usefulness of a 10% air-10% blood-80% saline mixture for contrast echocardiography: Doppler measurement of pulmonary artery systolic pressure. J Am Coll Cardiol 2002;39(1):124-9.

16. Mojadidi MK, Zhang L, Chugh Y, et al. Transcranial Doppler: does addition of blood to agitated saline Affect sensitivity for detecting cardiac right-to-left shunt? Echocardiography 2016;33(8):1219-27.

17. Droste DW, Lakemeier S, Wichter T, et al. Optimizing the technique of contrast transcranial Doppler ultrasound in the detection of right-to-left shunts. Stroke 2002;33(9):2211-6.

18. Johansson MC, Helgason H, Dellborg M, et al. Sensitivity for detection of patent foramen ovale increased with increasing number of contrast injections: a Descriptive study with contrast transesophageal echocardiography. J Am Soc Echocardiogr 2008;21(5):419-24.

19. Gin KG, Huckell VF, Pollick C. Femoral vein delivery of contrast medium enhances transthoracic echocardiographic detection of patent foramen ovale. J Am Coll Cardiol 1993;22(7):1994-2000.

20. Hamann GF, Schätzer-Klotz D, Fröhlig G, et al. Femoral injection of echo contrast medium may increase the sensitivity of testing for a patent foramen ovale. Neurology 1998;50(5):1423-8.

21. Saura D, García-Alberola A, Florenciano R, et al. Alternative explanations to the differences of femoral and brachial saline contrast injections for echocardiographic detection of patent foramen ovale. Med Hypotheses 2007;68(6):1378-81.

22. Gevorgyan R, Perlowski A, Shenoda M, et al. Sensitivity of brachial versus femoral vein injection of agitated saline to detect right-to-left shunts with Transcranial Doppler. Catheter Cardiovasc Interv 2014;84(6):992-6.

23. Sharma VK, Teoh HL, Chan BPL. Diagnosis of patent foramen ovale. JACC Cardiovasc Imaging 2010;3(10):1084.

24. Clarke NRA, Timperley J, Kelion AD, et al. Transthoracic echocardiography using second harmonic imaging with Valsalva manoeuvre for the detection of right to left shunts. Eur J Echocardiogr J Work Group Echocardiogr Eur Soc Cardiol 2004;5(3):176-81.

25. Mojadidi MK, Mahmoud AN, Elgendy IY, et al. Transesophageal echocardiography for the detection of patent foramen ovale. J Am Soc Echocardiogr 2017;30(9):933-4.

26. Di Tullio M, Sacco RL, Venketasubramanian N, et al. Comparison of diagnostic techniques for the detection of a patent foramen ovale in stroke patients. Stroke 1993;24(7):1020–4.

27. Japling MW, Kurowski JA, Williams SM. Patent foramen ovale— its correlation with other Maladies and a review of detection screening. US Neurol. 2015. Available at: https://touchneurology.com/headache-disorders/journal-articles/patent-foramen-ovale-its-correlation-with-other-maladies-and-a-review-of-detection-screening-2/. [Accessed 5 May 2023].

28. West BH, Noureddin N, Mamzhi Y, et al. The frequency of patent foramen ovale and migraine in patients with cryptogenic stroke. Stroke 2018;49(5):1123–8.

29. Lao AY, Sharma VK, Tsivgoulis G, et al. Detection of right-to-left shunts: comparison between the international consensus and Spencer logarithmic scale criteria. J Neuroimaging 2008;18(4):402–6.

30. Mojadidi MK, Winoker JS, Roberts SC, et al. Accuracy of conventional transthoracic echocardiography for the diagnosis of intracardiac right-to-left shunt: a meta-analysis of prospective studies. Echocardiography 2014;31(9):1036–48.

31. Mojadidi MK, Winoker JS, Roberts SC, et al. Two-dimensional echocardiography using second harmonic imaging for the diagnosis of intracardiac right-to-left shunt: a meta-analysis of prospective studies. Int J Cardiovasc Imaging 2014;30(5):911–23.

32. Katsanos AH, Psaltopoulou T, Sergentanis TN, et al. Transcranial Doppler versus transthoracic echocardiography for the detection of patent foramen ovale in patients with cryptogenic cerebral ischemia: a systematic review and diagnostic test accuracy meta-analysis. Ann Neurol 2016;79(4):625–35.

33. Scacciatella P, Meynet I, Giorgi M, et al. Angiography vs transesophageal echocardiography-guided patent foramen ovale closure: a propensity score matched analysis of a two-center registry. Echocardiography 2018;35(6):834–40.

34. Seiler C. How should we assess patent foramen ovale? Heart 2004;90(11):1245–7.

35. Overell JR, Bone I, Lees KR. Interatrial septal abnormalities and stroke: a meta-analysis of case-control studies. Neurology 2000;55(8):1172–9.

36. Mojadidi MK, Elgendy AY, Elgendy IY, et al. Transcatheter patent foramen ovale closure after cryptogenic stroke. JACC Cardiovasc Interv 2017;10(21):2228–30.

37. Wahl A, Meier B, Schwerzmann M, et al. Transcatheter treatment of atrial septal aneurysm associated with patent foramen ovale for prevention of recurrent paradoxical embolism in high-risk patients. J Am Coll Cardiol 2005;45(3):377–80.

38. Mojadidi MK, Ruiz JC, Chertoff J, et al. Patent foramen ovale and hypoxemia. Cardiol Rev 2019;27(1):34–40.

39. Schneider B, Zienkiewicz T, Jansen V, et al. Diagnosis of patent foramen ovale by transesophageal echocardiography and correlation with autopsy findings. Am J Cardiol 1996;77(14):1202–9.

40. Mojadidi MK, Bogush N, Caceres JD, et al. Diagnostic accuracy of transesophageal echocardiogram for the detection of patent foramen ovale: a meta-analysis. Echocardiography 2014;31(6):752–8.

41. Schuchlenz HW, Weihs W, Beitzke A, et al. Transesophageal echocardiography for quantifying size of patent foramen ovale in patients with cryptogenic Cerebrovascular events. Stroke 2002;33(1):293–6.

42. Bunch TJ, Day JD. Examining the risks and benefits of transesophageal echocardiogram imaging during catheter Ablation for atrial Fibrillation. Circ Arrhythm Electrophysiol 2012;5(4):621–3.

43. Rana BS, Thomas MR, Calvert PA, et al. Echocardiographic evaluation of patent foramen ovale prior to device closure. JACC Cardiovasc Imaging 2010;3(7):749–60.

44. Spencer MP, Moehring MA, Jesurum J, et al. Power M-mode transcranial Doppler for diagnosis of patent foramen ovale and assessing transcatheter closure. J Neuroimaging 2004;14(4):342–9.

45. Mojadidi MK, Roberts SC, Winoker JS, et al. Accuracy of transcranial Doppler for the diagnosis of intracardiac right-to-left shunt: a bivariate meta-analysis of prospective studies. JACC Cardiovasc Imaging 2014;7(3):236–50.

46. O'Brien MJ, Dorn AY, Ranjbaran M, et al. Fully Automated transcranial Doppler ultrasound for middle cerebral artery insonation. J Neurosonology Neuroimaging 2022;14(1):27–34.

47. Medford BA, Taggart NW, Cabalka AK, et al. Intracardiac echocardiography during atrial septal defect and patent foramen ovale device closure in Pediatric and Adolescent patients. J Am Soc Echocardiogr 2014;27(9):984–90.

48. Newton JD, Mitchell ARJ, Wilson N, et al. Intracardiac echocardiography for patent foramen ovale closure: Justification of routine Use. JACC Cardiovasc Interv 2009;2(4):369.

49. Hildick-Smith D, Behan M, Haworth P, et al. Patent foramen ovale closure without echocardiographic control: use of "Standby" intracardiac ultrasound. JACC Cardiovasc Interv 2008;1(4):387–91.

50. Van H, Poommipanit P, Shalaby M, et al. Sensitivity of transcranial Doppler versus intracardiac echocardiography in the detection of right-to-left shunt. JACC Cardiovasc Imaging 2010;3(4):343–8.

51. TEE versus ICE in Structural Interventions. American College of Cardiology. Available at: https://www.acc.org/latest-in-cardiology/articles/2018/09/10/08/09/http%3a%2f%2fwww.acc.org%2flatest-in-cardiology%2farticles%2f2018%2f09%2f10%2f08%2f09%2ftee-versus-ice-in-structural-interventions. [Accessed 5 November 2023].

52. Lüthy E, Rutishauser W, Hegglin R, et al. Über das Verhalten des arteriellen Sauerstoffgehaltes und der Farbstoff-Verdünnungskurven bei verschiedenen kongenitalen Vitien. Cardiology 1959;35(6):356–64.

53. Karttunen V, Ventilä M, Ikäheimo M, et al. Ear oximetry: a noninvasive method for detection of patent foramen ovale. Stroke 2001;32(2):448–53.

54. Billinger M, Schwerzmann M, Rutishauser W, et al. Patent foramen ovale screening by ear oximetry in Divers. Am J Cardiol 2013;111(2):286–90.

55. Devendra GP, Rane AA, Krasuski RA. Provoked Exercise desaturation in patent foramen ovale and Impact of percutaneous closure. JACC Cardiovasc Interv 2012;5(4):416–9.

56. Kim YJ, Hur J, Shim CY, et al. Patent foramen ovale: diagnosis with Multidetector CT—comparison with transesophageal echocardiography. Radiology 2009;250(1):61–7.

57. Kara K, Sivrioğlu AK, Öztürk E, et al. The role of coronary CT angiography in diagnosis of patent foramen ovale. Diagn Interv Radiol 2016;22(4):341–6.

58. Mohrs OK, Petersen SE, Erkapic D, et al. Dynamic contrast-enhanced MRI before and after transcatheter occlusion of patent foramen ovale. AJR Am J Roentgenol 2007;188(3):844–9.

59. Nusser T, Höher M, Merkle N, et al. Cardiac magnetic resonance imaging and transesophageal echocardiography in patients with transcatheter closure of patent foramen ovale. J Am Coll Cardiol 2006;48(2):322–9.

60. Mojadidi MK, Gevorgyan R, Tobis JM. A comparison of methods to detect and quantitate PFO: TCD, TTE, ICE and TEE. In: Amin Z, Tobis JM, Sievert H, et al, editors. Patent foramen ovale. Springer; 2015. p. 55–65. https://doi.org/10.1007/978-1-4471-4987-3_7.

Patent Foramen Ovale–Associated Stroke
A Neurologist's Perspective

Jeffrey L. Saver, MD

KEYWORDS

- Patent foramen ovale • Cryptogenic • Ischemic stroke • Diagnosis • Neurologist

KEY POINTS

- Paradoxic embolism through a patent foramen ovale (PFO) is a common cause of ischemic stroke, accounting for 1 in 20 of all ischemic strokes.
- Neurologists play the leading role in diagnosing PFO-associated stroke, determining that a cerebral infarct is embolic in distribution and excluding other potential stroke mechanisms.
- Among patients aged 18 to 60 years old with a PFO and an otherwise cryptogenic stroke, the PFO-Associated Stroke Causal Likelihood classification system should be used to identify the 85% of patients likely to benefit from PFO closure and the 15% of patients likely to be harmed by PFO closure.
- For young and middle-aged patients with PFO-associated stroke, moderate but important reductions in recurrent stroke can be achieved when neurologists and cardiologists collaboratively perform diagnostic evaluations and formulate therapeutic recommendations.

INTRODUCTION

Identifying paradoxic embolism through a patent foramen ovale (PFO) as a common, treatable cause of ischemic stroke is one of the great achievements of vascular neurology, in tandem with cardiology, in the last 40 years. The modern neurologic approach to the evaluation of ischemic stroke mechanisms was elaborated between the 1960s and 1980s and systematized in 1993 (in the Trial of Org 10,172 in Acute Stroke Treatment [TOAST] classification system). The TOAST system's ranking of the likeliness of different potential causes of stroke then remained unaltered for a remarkable 4 decades until accumulated epidemiologic and randomized clinical trial data mandated an update upgrading PFOs to status as a cardinal cause of cardioembolic ischemic stroke.[1] PFO-associated stroke is now recognized as the source of 5% of all ischemic strokes and a critical entity for understanding and management by neurologists, alongside cardiologists.[2]

CLINICAL EPIDEMIOLOGY

PFOs are found more commonly in patients with otherwise cryptogenic ischemic stroke than in patients with known-cause ischemic stroke. The degree of their increased frequency mathematically indicates how often they are actually causal of stroke. In the general population, PFOs are detected on transesophageal echocardiography (TEE) in 20% to 25% of individuals; atrial septal aneurysms (ASAs) are present in 2.2%, and 83% of patients with ASAs also have a PFO. In contrast, among young and middle-aged patients with cryptogenic ischemic stroke, PFOs are much more frequent, present in 50% to 60%. Meta-analysis of case-control studies comparing age-matched cryptogenic and known-cause stroke patients, corrected for potential publication bias, indicates that, among patients with otherwise cryptogenic ischemic stroke, in those under age 55 years, PFOs are present and causal in 38%, present but incidental in 13%, and absent in 48%.[2,3]

Department of Neurology and Comprehensive Stroke Center, David Geffen School of Medicine, University of California, Los Angeles, 710 Westwood Plaza, Los Angeles, CA 90095, USA
E-mail address: jsaver@mednet.ucla.edu

Cardiol Clin 42 (2024) 487–495
https://doi.org/10.1016/j.ccl.2024.01.006
0733-8651/24/© 2024 Elsevier Inc. All rights reserved.

cardiology.theclinics.com

Among those age 55 and older, PFOs are present and causal in 14%, present but incidental in 11%, and absent in 75%. These frequencies indicate that PFOs are a major cause of ischemic stroke and more common a source than low-burden atrial fibrillation (AF) (**Fig. 1**).[4] Overall, PFOs account for 5% of all cases, translating to 30,000 ischemic strokes per year in the United States and 575,000 ischemic strokes per year worldwide.

Diagnosis

General evaluation

The diagnostic evaluation of patients with ischemic stroke is a core competency of neurologists. All young and middle-aged ischemic stroke patients should undergo investigations to identify large artery atherosclerosis, cerebral small artery microatherosclerosis, nonatherosclerotic arteriopathies, structural and dysrhythmic cardiac sources of embolism, and arterial (and, if right-to-left shunt present, venous) hypercoagulable states.[5] The presence of a high-grade alternative source of stroke greatly lessens the likelihood that a medium-grade source like PFO is causative; and the presence of another medium-grade source reduces the likelihood to a lesser degree. Even when aortic, cervical, and cerebral vessel imaging has not identified substantial large artery atherosclerosis, the mere presence of risk factors for vascular disease, such as hypertension, hyperlipidemia, diabetes mellitus, and tobacco use, mildly diminishes the likelihood a detected PFO is causally related to the stroke.[6]

Embolic stroke topography

Analysis to determine if the distribution of an ischemic stroke is suggestive of an embolic rather than local thrombotic mechanism is a particularly distinctive contribution of neurologists to the assessment of the causal relatedness of a PFO. Emboli traversing the heart and arriving in the cerebral circulation tend to continue on a forward trajectory until reaching an artery too small to allow them to pass. Only uncommonly do they exit laminar flow streams at right angles to veer into a small deep-penetrating artery rather than continuing in the parent artery. As a result, embolic ischemic strokes are generally located superficially in the cerebrum.[7] If the emboli are small, they pass to very distal vessels and produce compact, superficial infarcts. If the emboli are large, they lodge in more proximal arteries and most often produce infarcts involving both superficial and deep regions. Less commonly the superficial region may be protected by robust collateral flow and large emboli will instead produce large, deep infarcts. Accordingly, infarcts involving superficial regions with or without deep regions and infarcts involving extensive deep regions are embolic in character, while infarcts involving a single, deep-penetrating artery ("lacunar" infarcts) are unlikely to be of embolic origin.

Patent foramen ovale detection and characterization

PFOs can be detected by transthoracic echocardiography (TTE), TEE, or transcranial Doppler ultrasound (TCD). Of these tests, TTE is the least sensitive, detecting only 50% to 60% of PFOs found on TEE or TCD. TEE and TCD have roughly equal sensitivities of ~90% and specificities greater than 95%. TCD detects 90% to 100% of

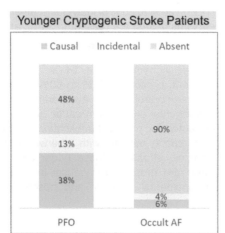
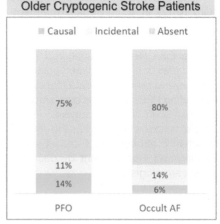

Fig. 1. Frequency and causal relatedness of (patent foramen ovale) PFO and occult atrial fibrillation (AF) among otherwise cryptogenic ischemic stroke patients. Left panel: Among younger patients: age less than 55 yo for PFO and age less than 65 yo for occult AF. Right panel: Among older patients: age ≥55 yo for PFO and age ≥65 yo for occult AF.

PFOs found on TEE and up to 10% missed with TEE; TCD may detect small PFOs missed by TEE in part as stronger Valsalva maneuvers can be elicited and confirmed to have occurred by change in TCD waveform, during TCD than TEE.[8] Conversely, TEE may detect small PFOs missed by TCD due to temporal bone thickening reducing the penetration of ultrasound to the middle cerebral artery. TEE and TCD are complementary. TEE, if tolerated by patients, uniquely characterizes PFO anatomy and presence of an ASA and assesses the presence of competing proximal sources of embolism, including aortic arch atherosclerosis, atrial appendage thrombi, and signs of atrial cardiopathy. TCD better quantifies PFO shunt size and uniquely detects spontaneous paradoxic microemboli that indicate higher imminent risk of stroke.

Venous thrombosis presence or disposition

A clinical history of circumstances promoting venous thrombosis suggests that a PFO is pathogenic rather than incidental, as they foster venous thromboemboli that may pass through the PFO. Recent immobility, such as extended plane or car travel, surgery, or illness, should be queried. Concomitant medical conditions predisposing to venous thrombosis include not only specific hypercoagulable states but also systemic malignancy, sepsis, chronic kidney disease, pregnancy, and known anatomic causes of venous congestion, such as May-Thurner syndrome. A personal past or family history of venous thromboembolism increases the risk. In addition, the history should determine if stroke onset occurred during or immediately after activities associated with a Valsalva maneuver that would have increased right-to-left shunting, including weightlifting, carrying luggage, playing a brass instrument, and straining at stool.

A comprehensive laboratory evaluation for a hypercoagulable state should be undertaken. Pure venous hypercoagulable states, such as protein C and S deficiencies, factor V Leiden mutation, and prothrombin gene mutation, increase the likelihood the PFO is causally related, as they foster venous thromboemboli that may pass through the PFO. In contrast, mixed arterial-venous hypercoagulable states, such as antiphospholipid antibodies or hyperhomocysteinemia, have bidirectional effects.[9] They promote both venous thromboemboli that may pass through the PFO but also arterial thrombi that may form in situ in the cerebral arterial tree, unrelated to the PFO.

The likelihood of PFO complicity in the ischemic stroke is strongly increased when concurrent deep or superficial venous thromboembolism is present on noninvasive lower extremity ultrasound, pelvic computed tomography or magnetic resonance venography, or pulmonary computed tomography arteriography performed within the first 48 to 72 hours after stroke onset (before time for venous thrombosis to develop secondarily).[10] Negative noninvasive testing by no means rules out a venous source—a substantial majority of venous clots are superficial (eg, calf) or small, deep thrombi discoverable only on invasive contrast venography.[11] However, invasive venography is uncomfortable for patients so it is not regularly obtained.

The patent foramen ovale–associated stroke causal likelihood diagnostic algorithm

Even in patients with otherwise cryptogenic strokes, a discovered PFO may be incidental rather than pathogenic. Consequently, a key further diagnostic step is to determine for each such patient the likelihood that their PFO was the source of their stroke using the clinical trial–validated logic algorithm PFO-Associated Stroke Causal Likelihood (PASCAL) classification system (**Fig. 2**).[12] Among patients with no major other defined cause of ischemic stroke, the PASCAL algorithm integrates information regarding (1) the presence of cardiac features that increase the likelihood of a PFO stroke mechanism (large shunt size and/or presence of an ASA) and (2) the absence of features that increase the likelihood of an occult non-PFO stroke mechanism as quantified in the Risk of Paradoxical Embolism score[6] (older age, non-embolic stroke topography, and vascular risk factors of hypertension, hyperlipidemia, diabetes mellitus, and tobacco use). Patients with both high-risk PFO features and a low burden of risk factors for a non-PFO stroke mechanism are classified as having *probable* PFO-associated strokes. Patients with either, but not both, high-risk PFO features and a low burden of risk factors for a non-PFO stroke mechanism are classified as having *possible* PFO-associated strokes. Lastly, patients with neither high-risk PFO features nor a low burden of risk factors for a non-PFO stroke mechanism are classified as having *unlikely* PFO-associated strokes. As detailed in the following therapeutic section, the PASCAL *probable* and *possible* categories identify patients who will experience net benefit from PFO closure while the PASCAL *unlikely* category identifies patients who will experience net harm from PFO closure. Among patients enrolled in randomized clinical trials of PFO closure, the frequencies of each PASCAL subtype were *probable*—37%, *possible*—48%, *unlikely*—15%.

High Risk PFO Features **Present** *Large Shunt +/or ASA*	Risk Factors for non-PFO Mechanism **Absent** *RoPE Score ≥ 7*	PFO Causal Relation
✓	✓	PROBABLE
✓	X	POSSIBLE
X	✓	
X	X	Unlikely

Fig. 2. The Patent Foramen Ovale–Associated Stroke Causal Likelihood (PASCAL) classification system to determine patent foramen ovale (PFO) causal likelihood.

EVIDENTIAL BASIS FOR TREATMENT
Best Medical Therapy

Among antithrombotic agents, physiologic reasoning suggests that anticoagulation might be superior to antiplatelet therapy, as anticoagulants better avert the stasis thrombi that arise in veins. However, anticoagulation is also associated with increased bleeding and comparative studies are only weakly suggestive of an efficacy advantage. The 2 randomized trials that have head-to-head compared anticoagulant against antiplatelet therapy in subgroups of patients with PFOs and cryptogenic ischemic strokes found nonsignificant efficacy differences favoring anticoagulation: PICSS trial (PFO in Cryptogenic Stroke Study; hazard ratio [HR], 0.52; 95% confidence interval [CI], 0.16–1.67; $P = .28$)[13] and CLOSE trial (Patent Foramen Ovale Closure or Anticoagulants vs Antiplatelet Therapy to Prevent Stroke Recurrence; HR, 0.44; 95% CI, 0.11–1.48; $P = .18$).[14] Conversely, minor bleeding complications were significantly and major bleeding complications were nominally more frequent among anticoagulated patients. Additional modest support for superiority of anticoagulation in averting ischemic stroke is provided by an individual participant data meta-analysis of 12 prospective observational studies and randomized trials also nonsignificantly favoring anticoagulation compared with antiplatelet therapy (HR, 0.75; 95% CI, 0.44–1.27).[15] Compared with older anticoagulants, newer, direct oral anticoagulants (DOACs) are promising options, with more predictable blood levels and reduced bleeding rates. In a meta-analysis of trials in patients with deep vein thrombosis (DVT), DOACs were equivalent to warfarin in averting recurrent venous thromboembolism and superior in avoiding bleeding complications.[16] However, randomized trials of DOACs in patients with PFO-associated stroke have not been conducted.

Best Endovascular Device Therapy

Percutaneously placed PFO closure devices resolve the potential for recurrent paradoxic embolism by permanently anatomically closing the interatrial passage. Closure device designs differ in important ways that affect ease of delivery, efficacy in achieving complete closure, and adverse effects. Devices tested in randomized trials may be grouped into 2 broad classes, based on frame shape: the first generation of devices had umbrella-clamshell contours, with some frame projection away from the septal surface, whereas later developed devices had double-disk contours, a more compact profile potentially less prone to complications.[17] In a randomized trial directly comparing 3 closure devices against one another, including 1 umbrella-clamshell device (CardioSEAL STARflex occluder [C]) and 2 double-disk devices (Amplatzer PFO occluder [A] and HELEX occluder [H]), better outcomes were observed with the double-disk devices, including fewer recurrent ischemic events (A, 1.4%; H, 4.1%; C, 5.9%), less thrombosis on device (A, 0.0%; H, 0.5%; C, 5.0%), and less AF (A, 3.6%; H, 2.3%; C, 12.3%).[18]

Endovascular Versus Medical Therapy

PFO closure devices and medical therapy have been compared in 6 randomized trials, collectively enrolling 3740 patients with PFOs and otherwise cryptogenic ischemic strokes who were followed for a median of 4 years 9 months.[2,12] All enrolled young or middle-aged stroke patients, primarily of ages 18 to 60, with a median age of 46 (interquartile range 39–53). In the medical arm, antiplatelet agents were most commonly employed, accounting for more than 86% of patient-years of therapy; the remaining medical patients who were treated with anticoagulation were predominantly on warfarin rather than DOACs. In the device arm, 5 of the trials tested double-disk devices (the Amplatzer PFO occluder or the Gore Helex device) and 1 trial tested a clamshell device.

Efficacy

Overall, individual participant data pooled analysis of all 6 randomized trials showed a highly statistically significant and moderately clinically significant advantage of device therapy in averting recurrent ischemic stroke (**Table 1**).[12] In relative terms, the magnitude of the treatment effect was substantial. The rate of any recurrent ischemic stroke was reduced by more than half and the rate of recurrent ischemic stroke with only PFO as an identified cause was reduced by more than three-quarters. Disabling recurrent ischemic stroke also showed a nonsignificant more than 40% relative reduction. In absolute terms, both treatment groups did fairly well, with low recurrent event rates, but the device group did better. At 2 years, about 5.5% of medical patients had a recurrent ischemic stroke compared with 2.4% of device patients. The number needed to treat to avert 1 stroke over 5 years was 32.

The trials also provided important information on technical efficacy in achieving PFO closure. After device placement, there was effective PFO closure (no or only trace residual shunting) in 93% to 96% of patients in double-disk trials and in 87% in the umbrella-clamshell trial.[2]

Safety

Serious, immediate, procedure-related complications were infrequent among the 1780 of 1889 patients allocated to the device groups who actually underwent a placement procedures and included access site or retroperitoneal hemorrhage in 1.01%, pericardial tamponade in 0.17%, and cardiac perforation in 0.06%.[2]

The most common complication of device placement was AF. Overall AF occurred in 5.0% of device patients compared with 1.1% of control patients.[12] But the great preponderance of AF events were transient episodes occurring in the first 4 to 6 weeks after device placement, during the first settling of device elements into atrial tissue, which have less likelihood of serving as a new stroke source. Late only-onset AF beyond the periprocedural period showed a nonsignificant 0.39% annual increase in AF with closure in the double-disk device trials with available data.[2] Venous thromboembolism was infrequent but

higher in the device group, 1.4% versus 0.5% over the entire follow-up period, likely reflecting the less frequent use of anticoagulation in device patients.[12]

Modification of Treatment Effect in Patient Subgroups

Individual patient features

Among individual patient characteristics, the most notable modifiers of treatment benefit are the presence of cardiac features potentiating PFO risk: large shunt size and ASA (**Fig. 3**).[19] If neither was present, device placement did not statistically alter recurrent stroke rates. If either was present alone, device placement showed modest benefit, reducing recurrent stroke rates by 2% to 2.5% over 5 years. However, if both high-risk features were present, device placement showed substantial benefit, reducing recurrent stroke rates by 7.1% over 5 years.

Patent foramen ovale–associated stroke causal likelihood probable, possible, and unlikely levels

The PASCAL classification system showed strong effect modification, with both efficacy and safety increasing across the 3 classification levels (**Fig. 4**).[12,20] For efficacy as assessed by recurrent stroke, among PASCAL *probable* patients, HRs were reduced dramatically, by 90%, in device patients. Among PASCAL *possible* patients, HRs were reduced substantially, by 62%, in device patients. In contrast, among PASCAL *unlikely* patients, no statistical differences were noted and the point estimate for recurrent stroke was actually 14% higher in the device group.

The safety outcome of AF showed a contrasting pattern. Among PASCAL *probable* patients, absolute rates of new-onset AF beyond the periprocedural period were not significantly increased in device patients, with point estimate of 0.7% higher. Among PASCAL *possible* patients, late AF onset increase in device patients was moderate, 1.5%

Table 1
Device versus medical therapy recurrent stroke prevention in randomized trials

Outcome	Events per 100 Person-Years		Absolute Difference at 2y	Relative Risk, Adjusted	
	Device	Medical		HR (95% CI)	P Value
Any recurrent ischemic stroke	0.47	1.09	1.7%	0.41 (0.28–0.60)	<.001
PFO-associated recurrent ischemic stroke	0.24	0.90	2.2%	0.24 (0.14–0.43)	<.001
Disabling recurrent ischemic stroke	0.16	0.27	0.2%	0.59 (0.37–1.22)	.14

Abbreviations: CI, confidence interval; HR, hazard ratio; PFO, patent foramen ovale.

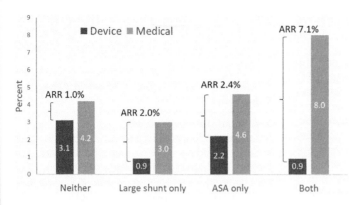

Fig. 3. Modification of patent foramen ovale (PFO) closure benefit in reducing recurrent ischemic stroke over 5 years by the presence of large shunt size, atrial septal aneurysm (ASA), or both.

higher. In contrast, among PASCAL *unlikely* patients, late AF onset increase among device patients was substantially increased, by 4.4%.

This pattern of escalating benefit and decreasing harm across the 3 PA levels accords with pathophysiologic expectations. The more likely the index stroke is due to the PFO, the greater the expected reduction in recurrent stroke by PFO closure. Conversely, the less likely the index stroke is due to the PFO, the more likely it was due to undiagnosed occult AF that would be exacerbated by device placement.

These findings have important clinical implications. Both PASCAL *probable* and PASCAL *possible* patients experience net benefit from device placement, with magnitude of recurrent stroke reduction substantially larger than magnitude of AF increase. However, PASCAL *unlikely* patients may experience net harm from device

placement, with the magnitude of recurrent stroke reduction smaller than magnitude of AF increase.

Effect modification by medical therapy strategy
Among the 3 trials with separately reported medical therapy treatment subgroups, there was evidence of heterogeneity of treatment effect depending on the type of medical antithrombotic therapy employed in the medical group.[2] Compared with medical antiplatelet therapy alone, device closure was superior in averting recurrent stroke (HR, 0.19; 95% CI, 0.06–0.56). In contrast, in the underpowered comparison of medical therapy with anticoagulants alone versus device closure plus long-term antiplatelet therapy, no benefit of device closure was noted (HR, 1.32; 95% CI, 0.43–4.03).

Is the effect magnitude clinically worthwhile?
During the follow-up in randomized trials, the benefit magnitude of PFO closure was overall moderate, but higher in select patients and generally in a range likely to be deemed clinically worthwhile by a substantial proportion of patients and families. But it is important to recognize that the less than 5 year average follow-up in randomized clinical trials is likely to be conservative with regard to benefit estimate. Young and middle-aged ischemic stroke patients with PFO and first cryptogenic ischemic stroke have decades of future at-risk years. Modest annual reductions in stroke rates, if sustained, have many years to additively accrue value. Further, these estimates may also be conservative due to a bias in the type of patients enrolled in the trials. Some patients with perceived high recurrence risk on medical therapy were likely treated with device closure outside the trials, rather than enrolled and randomized.

The annual recurrent ischemic stroke reduction is modest is that event rates in patients treated

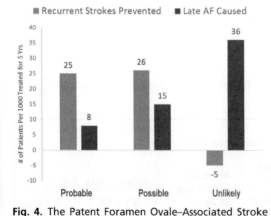

Fig. 4. The Patent Foramen Ovale–Associated Stroke Causal Likelihood (PASCAL) classification system and patent foramen ovale (PFO) closure benefit and harm. Among 1000 patients over 5 years of follow-up, the number of recurrent strokes prevented (*green*) and new onset of post-periprocedural atrial fibrillation caused (*red*).

with medical therapy alone are low to start with, 1.2% per year across the 6 randomized controlled trials (RCTs), placing a ceiling on how much further benefit device placement can confer. This low recurrence rate on medical therapy is less than with other causes of stroke and accords with the status of PFOs as medium-grade, not high-grade, risk sources for stroke, less menacing than severe carotid stenosis or chronic AF. Consequently, patients have a welcome choice between 2 good treatment options—medical therapy alone, with a modest recurrence rate, or closure, with a dramatic relative, and moderate absolute, further reduction in risk.

SUMMARY

Paradoxic embolism through a PFO is a common cause of ischemic stroke, accounting for 1 in 20 of all ischemic strokes. Neurologists play the leading role in diagnosing PFO-Associated stroke, determining that a cerebral infarct is embolic in distribution and excluding other potential stroke mechanisms. Among patients aged 18 to 60 year old with a PFO and an otherwise cryptogenic stroke, the PASCAL classification system should be used to identify the 85% of patients likely to benefit from PFO closure and the 15% of patients likely to be harmed by PFO closure. The benefit of PFO closure in patients over age 60 is uncertain, but likely to be present for physiologically younger individuals who are age 61 to 65 and perhaps older. For young and middle-aged patients with PFO-associated stroke, moderate but important reductions in recurrent stroke can be achieved when neurologists and cardiologists collaboratively perform diagnostic evaluations and formulate therapeutic recommendations.

CLINICAL CARE POINTS

For patients aged 18 to 60 years

- Young and middle-aged otherwise cryptogenic stroke patients with PFO should know that both medical therapy and device therapy are good choices for most patients. Recurrence rates are low with antiplatelet therapy alone, potentially lower with anticoagulation therapy alone, and definitely lower with device therapy.
- Patients with both a large shunt and an ASA are at an especially magnified risk of recurrent stroke on medical therapy and generally should be treated with closure.

- Among the remaining otherwise cryptogenic stroke patients with PFO, the PASCAL classification algorithm should be deployed to inform treatment decisions.
  - PFO closure should be strongly considered in patients classified as having index strokes of *probable* or *possible* PFO origin as they will experience net benefit (reduced recurrent stroke) from device placement.
  - PFO closure should generally be avoided in patients classified as having index strokes of *unlikely* PFO origin as they will experience net harm (no stroke reduction and substantially increased AF) from device placement.
- In patients with a history of overt DVT, and possibly patients with venous hypercoagulable states, long-term anticoagulation with or without device placement is indicated to avert DVT and pulmonary embolism, as well as recurrent ischemic stroke.
- In patients in whom anticoagulation is contraindicated due to past bleeding complications or bleeding prone conditions, device placement is preferred. Similarly, for patients in whom frequent or prolonged interruption of oral anticoagulation may be anticipated, because of multiple surgical or invasive procedures, pregnancy, or medication nonadherence, device placement is an attractive option.
- Closing the PFO will prevent future PFO-related strokes, but not strokes due to other causes. As the diagnosis of PFO-associated stroke is almost always probabilistic rather than definitive, the possibility of an alternative stroke mechanism as the actual culprit cannot generally be completely excluded. Accordingly, it is reasonable to treat patients who undergo device closure with lifelong low-dose antiplatelet therapy as well, rather than discontinuing all antithrombotic agents after device endothelialization, to provide ongoing protection against unrecognized possible competing causes of the initial stroke.

For patients over age 60

- Older patients are more likely to harbor competing, low-to-medium risk potential causes of the index stroke, reducing the likelihood that an identified PFO is causally related to the cryptogenic stroke.[3]
- But older individuals are also more prone to venous thromboembolism,[21] and those with a PFO are prone to more right-to-left shunting, in part because of a higher prevalence of sleep apnea, increasing the likelihood that a discovered PFO is causally related to the cryptogenic stroke.

- Also, older individuals may be more prone to the complication of closure device–induced AF.
- Given these age-related differences, RCTs in individuals over age 60 are needed. Pending those studies, PFO device closure might be deployed highly selectively, especially in younger old patients, ages 61 to 65, and after more extensive workup for paroxysmal AF, with at least 4 weeks of ambulatory monitoring.

Systems of care

- At the systems level, the management of patients with PFO and cryptogenic stroke requires close coordination between neurologists and cardiologists expert in the evaluation and treatment of neuro-cardiovascular diseases. An emerging model is a jointly run specialized outpatient clinic at which cryptogenic stroke patients, with or without PFO, can be efficiently evaluated by both specialties.[22]
- Neurologists' insights on distinctive features of the stroke presentation and topography, and cardiologists' insights on distinctive features of the PFO anatomy and other cardiac structural and rhythm findings, can be synthesized into an integrated perspective on likely stroke mechanism and likely benefits and risks of the different therapeutic options for consideration by patients and families.

DISCLOSURE

J.L. Saver has received, for service on clinical trial steering committees and DSMBs advising on rigorous study design and conduct, hourly payments from Abbott and Occlutech.

REFERENCES

1. Elgendy AY, Saver JL, Amin Z, et al. Proposal for updated Nomenclature and classification of potential causative mechanism in patent foramen ovale-associated stroke. JAMA Neurol 2020;77:878–86.
2. Saver JL, Mattle HP, Thaler D. Patent foramen ovale closure versus medical therapy for cryptogenic ischemic stroke: a Topical Review. Stroke 2018;49:1541–8.
3. Alsheikh-Ali AA, Thaler DE, Kent DM. Patent foramen ovale in cryptogenic stroke: incidental or pathogenic? Stroke 2009;40:2349–55.
4. Chaisinanunkul N, Khurshid S, Buck BH, et al. How often is occult atrial fibrillation in cryptogenic stroke causal vs. incidental? A meta-analysis. Front Neurol 2023;14:1103664.
5. Saver JL. Cryptogenic stroke. N Engl J Med 2016;374:2065–74.
6. Kent DM, Ruthazer R, Weimar C, et al. An index to identify stroke-related vs incidental patent foramen ovale in cryptogenic stroke. Neurology 2013;81:619–25.
7. Sharobeam A, Churilov L, Parsons M, et al. Patterns of infarction on MRI in patients with Acute ischemic stroke and Cardio-embolism: a systematic Review and meta-analysis. Available at: Front Neurol 2020;11 https://www.frontiersin.org/articles/10.3389/fneur.2020.606521. [Accessed 11 December 2023].
8. Mojadidi MK, Bogush N, Caceres JD, et al. Diagnostic accuracy of transesophageal echocardiogram for the detection of patent foramen ovale: a meta-analysis. Echocardiography 2014;31:752–8.
9. Carroll BJ, Piazza G. Hypercoagulable states in arterial and venous thrombosis: when, how, and who to test? Vasc Med 2018;23:388–99.
10. Lapergue B, Decroix JP, Evrard S, et al. Diagnostic Yield of venous thrombosis and pulmonary embolism by Combined CT venography and pulmonary Angiography in patients with cryptogenic stroke and patent foramen ovale. Eur Neurol 2015;74:69–72.
11. Lethen H, Flachskampf FA, Schneider R, et al. Frequency of deep vein thrombosis in patients with patent foramen ovale and ischemic stroke or transient ischemic attack. Am J Cardiol 1997;80:1066–9.
12. Kent DM, Saver JL, Kasner SE, et al. Heterogeneity of treatment effects in an analysis of pooled individual patient data from randomized trials of device closure of patent foramen ovale after stroke. JAMA 2021;326:2277–86.
13. Homma S, Sacco RL, Di Tullio MR, et al. PFO in Cryptogenic Stroke Study (PICSS) Investigators. Effect of medical treatment in stroke patients with patent foramen ovale: patent foramen ovale in Cryptogenic Stroke Study. Circulation 2002;105:2625–31.
14. Mas J-L, Derumeaux G, Guillon B, et al. Patent foramen ovale closure or anticoagulation vs. Antiplatelets after stroke. N Engl J Med 2017;377:1011–21.
15. Kent DM, Dahabreh IJ, Ruthazer R, et al. Anticoagulant vs. antiplatelet therapy in patients with cryptogenic stroke and patent foramen ovale: an individual participant data meta-analysis. Eur Heart J 2015;36:2381–9.
16. Wang X, Ma Y, Hui X, et al. Oral direct thrombin inhibitors or oral factor Xa inhibitors versus conventional anticoagulants for the treatment of deep vein thrombosis. Cochrane Database Syst Rev 2023;4:CD010956.
17. Nassif M, Abdelghani M, Bouma BJ, et al. Historical developments of atrial septal defect closure devices: what we learn from the past. Expert Rev Med Devices 2016;13:555–68.
18. Hornung M, Bertog SC, Franke J, et al. Long-term results of a randomized trial comparing three

different devices for percutaneous closure of a patent foramen ovale. Eur Heart J 2013;34: 3362–9.

19. Mas J-L, Saver JL, Kasner SE, et al. Association of atrial septal aneurysm and shunt size with stroke recurrence and benefit from patent foramen ovale closure. JAMA Neurol 2022;79:1175–9.

20. Termeie O, Saver JL, Kasner SE, et al. PFO Closure to Avert Recurrent Stroke: The PASCAL Stratification System Distinguishes Patient Groups with Net Benefit and Net Harm. Munich: 2023.

21. Heit JA. Epidemiology of venous thromboembolism. Nat Rev Cardiol 2015;12:464–74.

22. Immens MH, van den Hoeven V, van Lith TJ, et al. Heart-Stroke Team: a multidisciplinary assessment of patent foramen ovale-associated stroke. European Stroke Journal 2023. https://doi.org/10.1177/23969873231214862.

Migraine Headache and Patent Foramen Ovale

Observational Studies, the Randomized Clinical Trials, and the GORE RELIEF Clinical Study

Robert J. Sommer, MD[a],*, Barbara T. Robbins, FNP-BC[a]

KEYWORDS

• Patent foramen ovale • Migraine headache • Trials • Platelets • P2Y12 inhibition

KEY POINTS

• The underlying pathophysiology of migraines remains poorly defined.
• In some patients, the right-to-left shunt associated with patent foramen ovale (PFO) seems to be a critical component in the initiation of migraines.
• Early trials of PFO closure for migraine failed in part due to the inability to distinguish PFOs, which were mechanistically linked to migraines ("causal" PFO) from those that were simply coincidental to the migraines.
• In order to truly assess the magnitude of the benefit of PFO closure for migraines or successfully run a trial to demonstrate such a benefit, researchers will need to be able to identify and treat only the causal PFO patients.
• The use of platelet P2Y12 inhibition therapy as a test for PFO causality may allow us to demonstrate the efficacy of PFO closure in a subset of migraine patients. This concept is being studied in the GORE RELIEF Clinical Study which is currently enrolling.

BACKGROUND

Migraine headache (MHA) is the most prevalent neurologic disorder in humans and the leading cause of disease-related disability among young and middle-aged adults.[1,2] It is also one of the oldest ailments known to mankind.[3] The Egyptians documented cases of painful headaches as far back as 1200 BC. Preceding visual aura was first described by Hippocrates in 400 BC, and recurrent unilateral headaches associated with vomiting and light sensitivity were first described in detail by Aretaeus of Cappadocia in the second century AD.

Therapy to prevent migraine, however, is far more recent. Prior to the 1960s, the treatment of migraine was limited to acute headache relief. But with the introduction of beta-blockers,[4] developed for the prevention of anginal pain, some patients with a prior history of migraine noted an unexpected reduction in headache frequency and severity while taking the medication. Later, other medications, calcium-channel blockers for hypertension,[5] onabotulinumtoxin A for cosmetic dermatologic therapy,[6,7] valproate and topiramate for seizure prevention,[8] candesartan for hypertension,[9] and amitriptyline and selective serotonin reuptake inhibitors for depression[10] were all unexpectedly found to have similar beneficial effects in some migraine sufferers. Most recently, calcitonin gene-related peptide (CGRP) was implicated as a critical messenger in migraine pain signaling in the trigeminal nerve distribution of the head and neck.[11]

[a] Department of Medicine, Division of Interventional Cardiology, Columbia University Medical Center, 161 Fort Washington Avenue, Room 624, New York, NY 10032, USA
* Corresponding author.
E-mail address: rs2463@cumc.columbia.edu

Cardiol Clin 42 (2024) 497–507
https://doi.org/10.1016/j.ccl.2024.01.007
0733-8651/24/© 2024 Elsevier Inc. All rights reserved.

Anti-CGRP antibodies introduced in 2018 and anti-CGRP receptor antibodies approved in 2021 as the first migraine-specific preventive therapies have made significant contributions in some patients. Our lack of understanding of migraine pathophysiology is underscored by the fact that this wide array of drugs, for disparate disease states, is all being used for migraine prevention and that none of these treatments, including the CGRP inhibitors, work for all migraineurs.

The classic migraine "attack" involves a complex cascade of physiologic events involving cerebral vasoconstriction/hypoperfusion followed by vasodilation/hyperemia, an associated sterile inflammation, and hypersensitization of pain receptors particularly in the trigeminal nerve distribution.[12] Each of the migraine preventives may work to interrupt specific aspects of these pathways. It is not known why some therapies work for some patients and others do not but this may be related to the relative contribution of each aspect of the migraine cycle in the individual patient. As an alternative theory, there may be a variety of patient-specific underlying physiologic mechanisms which trigger the onset of the attack. Ideally, if testing was available to identify these mechanisms, each patient could be treated with directed/personalized therapy rather than the current trial-and-error approach.

INITIAL OBSERVATIONS

The association between MHAs and patent foramen ovale (PFO) began with observations in the 1990s that migraine sufferers, particularly those with aura, were more likely to have thromboembolic stroke. In early work, Tzourio and colleagues[13] demonstrated an independent risk between migraine and the risk for ischemic stroke in a French case-controlled study. Henrich and Horwitz[14] performed a prospective hospital-based, case-controlled study comparing migraineurs and non-migraineurs and demonstrated a strong and significant association between migraine and ischemic stroke.

Since the association between stroke and PFO had been strongly established by that time,[15,16] it did not take long for observational population studies to recognize an increased PFO prevalence in the migraine population, specifically in those suffering migraine with aura. Anzola and colleagues, in a transcranial Doppler study, found that the prevalence of PFO in migraine/aura patients was twice that of either migraine/no aura patients or non-migraine controls.[17] In a meta-analysis of 6 PFO/migraine studies, Schwedt and colleagues[18] demonstrated that the presence of a PFO was 5 times as likely in migraine patients than in non-migraine controls (**Fig. 1**A) and that the prevalence of migraines was 2.5 times as great in patients with PFO than in patients with intact atrial septum (**Fig. 1**B). Again, the greatest association was between PFO and migraine/aura.

While the pathophysiologic mechanism linking PFO to migraine was unknown, it was assumed to be related to the right-to-left shunt associated with PFO, as other types of patients with right-to-left shunts, such as those with cyanotic congenital heart disease[19] and those with Osler–Weber–Rendu syndrome[20] (now hereditary hemorrhagic telangiectasia) with pulmonary arteriovenous malformations, were also demonstrated to have a significantly higher incidence of migraine/aura than the general population.

By the late 1990s, application of transcatheter PFO closure had become widespread for the prevention of recurrent stroke. Wilmshurst and colleagues,[21] in a paper in 2000, described the first series of patients with unexpected migraine

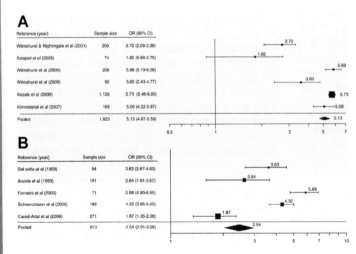

Fig. 1. (*A*) Strength of association between patent foramen ovale (PFO) and migraine. The odds ratios (ORs) for migraine and PFO ranged from 1.82 to 5.88, with a summary OR of 5.13 [95% confidence interval (CI) 4.67–5.59]. (*B*) Strength of association between migraine and patent foramen ovale (PFO). The ORs ranged from 1.87 to 5.88, with a summary OR of 2.54 [95% CI 2.01–3.08]. (*From* Schwedt TJ, Demaerschalk BM & Dodicl DW. Patent foramen ovale and migraine: a quantitative systematic review. Cephalagia 2008; 28:531-540.)

elimination following PFO closure performed for other reasons. This was followed by a series of retrospective/observational papers reporting MHA reduction of 57% to 91% following PFO closure for secondary stroke prevention.[22–30]

THE EARLY MIGRAINE–PATENT FORAMEN OVALE TRIALS

These observational series generated tremendous excitement and led to the design of 4 clinical trials in the early 2000s to test the hypothesis that PFO closure was an effective therapy for migraine.

The MIST trial[31] was published in 2008. The trial included only patients having migraine with aura, who experienced ≥5 migraine days per month with at least 7 headache-free days per month (episodic migraine), who had previously failed 2 classes of prophylactic treatments, and who had moderate or large right-to-left shunts consistent with the presence of a PFO. These subjects were randomized to either transcatheter PFO closure with the CardioSEAL STARFlex Septal Occluder (NMT Medical, Boston, MA; **Fig. 2**) or to a sham catheter procedure. The primary efficacy end point was cessation of MHA at 6 months after the catheter procedure. One hundred forty-seven patients were randomized. There was no difference in the primary efficacy end point between the implant and the sham cohorts (3/74 vs 3/73). Secondary end points also failed to reach statistical significance.

The ESCAPE Migraine Trial[32] was discontinued prior to completing enrollment. This study also focused on patients with episodic headaches who had failed conventional therapy. In an effort to select the most appropriate patients for PFO closure with the PREMERE PFO Occluder (St. Jude Medical Inc, St. Paul, MN; **Fig. 3**), the inclusion/exclusion

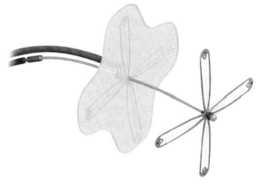

Fig. 3. The PREMERE PFO Occluder (Abbott, Abbott 'A', Premere are trademarks of Abbott or its related companies. Reproduced with permission of Abbott, © 2024. All rights reserved.).

criteria were so onerous that the participating neurologist investigators reported needing to screen more than 100 patients to identify a single eligible subject. The trial was closed after fewer than 30 subjects were enrolled over a period of 3 years.

The PRIMA Trial[33] enrolled its first subject in 2006. Enrollment was halted short of the expected cohort size after 107 subjects were enrolled by 2012. Subjects included only migraineurs with aura, who had episodic migraines and had failed 2 traditional migraine preventatives. Treatment was randomized 1:1 to either PFO closure with the Amplatzer PFO Occluder (Abbott Cardiovascular, Plymouth, MN; **Fig. 4**) or to on-going

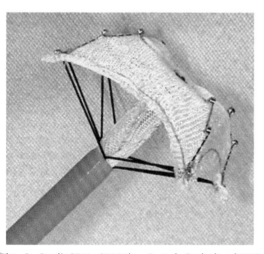

Fig. 2. CardioSEAL STARFlex Septal Occluder (NMT Medical, Boston, MA).

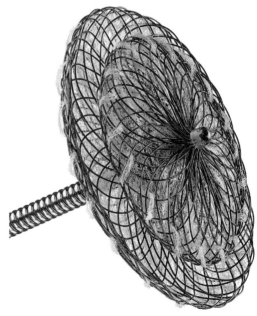

Fig. 4. The Amplatzer PFO Occluder (Abbott, Abbott 'A', Amplatzer are trademarks of Abbott or its related companies. Reproduced with permission of Abbott, © 2024. All rights reserved.).

medical therapy and as such was unblinded. Only 41 of 53 subjects randomized to the device arm actually received a device. Eight withdrew consent prior to the catheter procedure and no PFO was identified at catheterization in another 4 subjects; 40 of 41 subjects in the device cohort completed the 12 month follow-up and 43 of 54 subjects who were assigned to the medical arm completed the 12 month follow-up. The primary end point reduction in monthly migraine days at 1 year after randomization was not met based on an intent-to-treat analysis. The mean reduction of migraine days per month was greater in the PFO closure group but was not statistically significant (P = .17).

The PREMIUM trial[34] also began enrollment in 2006 and completed enrollment 7 years later. Inclusion criteria allowed both migraine with aura and migraine without aura but excluded patients with chronic migraine (>15 headache days/month) and patients with fewer than 6 headache days per month. All subjects had failed at least 3 preventative therapies. Two hundred thirty subjects were randomized to either PFO closure with the Amplatzer PFO Occluder (N = 123) or to a sham catheterization procedure (N = 107). Catheterization laboratory treatment was blinded for both the subject and the treating neurologist; 119 of 123 subjects had a successful PFO device implant of whom 117 reached the designated 12 month trial conclusion and 103 of 107 sham subjects completed the 12-month follow-up. The primary efficacy end point, the "Responder Rate," was defined as the frequency of subjects who had at least a 50% reduction in migraine attacks after percutaneous closure of PFO with the Amplatzer PFO Occluder. The primary efficacy end point was not met; 38.5% in the device arm and 32% of the sham subjects had a 50% reduction in migraine attacks (P = .32). Two secondary efficacy end points were met. There was a significant decrease in the mean number of migraine days per month in the device versus the sham groups: −3.4 ± 4.4 days versus −2.0 ± 5.0 days (P = .025), and there was a significant difference in subjects who had complete cessation of migraine attacks: 8.5% in the device arm versus 1.0% in the sham cohort (P = .01). Of these, 6 subjects had had frequent migraine aura, while 4 subjects had no history of aura.

A subsequent meta-analysis of the PRIMA and PREMIUM trials was performed by Mojadidi and colleagues.[35] In this analysis, 337 subjects from the 2 trials were pooled (176 who had undergone PFO closure and 161 who had medical treatment alone). Because the original studies had different primary end points, the authors redefined the analysis to include all 4 end points from the 2 trials. In addition to the frequency of patients attaining a 50% reduction in monthly migraines, the investigators also assessed reduction in monthly headache days, reduction in monthly migraine attacks (some spanned more than 1 day), and complete cessation of migraine activity. Three of the four endpoints were met (**Fig. 5**) with statistically significant reductions in both monthly migraine days and migraine attacks in the PFO closure cohort compared with the control group. Complete migraine elimination occurred 9 times as often in the PFO closure group. While the metanalysis demonstrated a statistical migraine benefit to PFO closure for the first time, like with any metanalysis there were significant limitations inherent to the retrospective pooling of patient cohorts that were not entirely comparable and to fundamental methodological differences such as subjects being blinded in the PREMIUM trial but not in PRIMA.

WHY DID THE EARLY PATENT FORAMEN OVALE–MIGRAINE TRIALS FAIL?

Part of the explanation for the trial failures was that the early PFO-migraine trials were small and may have lacked the statistical power to demonstrate small clinical differences. But the more fundamental issue, common to all PFO-migraine trials to date, was the lack of understanding of the underlying pathophysiologic mechanisms linking the migraines to the PFO. The designers of the original trials recognized that 25% of migraineurs had a PFO. That defined the other 75% of the population as having a "non-PFO" migraine mechanism. The unstated assumption of the early trials was that the PFO was mechanistically linked ("causal") in all of the migraineurs who had one. But as worldwide experience and clinical trials have shown, just like with other migraine therapies, some migraine patients simply do not benefit from PFO closure. Because of the prevalence of PFO in the general population, it is nearly certain that some of these migraine patients would have had a non-PFO migraine mechanism but would also have had a PFO. Closure of these "incidental" PFOs would produce no migraine benefit, and their inclusion in any trial would confound not only the statistical analysis but also any potential understanding of the true benefit of the treatment.

Similarly, we cannot be sure that the assumptions made in the trials to help enrich the patient population were a help or a hindrance to the study outcomes. For example, 3 of the 4 trials included only patients with migraine/aura, but the PREMIUM Study showed that a significant number of patients without aura also responded to PFO closure. The trials allowed only patients with

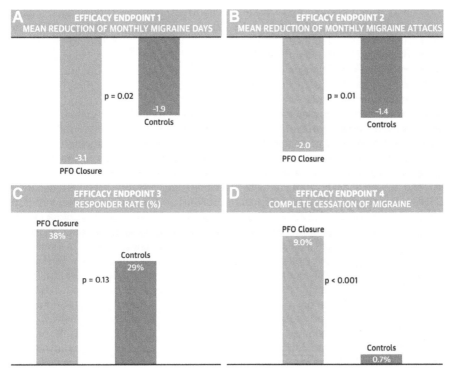

Fig. 5. Compared with control subjects, patent foramen ovale (PFO) closure yielded a significant mean reduction of monthly migraine days, a mean reduction of monthly migraine attacks, and a greater number of patients with complete migraine cessation ($P \leq .05$ for all). There was no significant difference in the responder rate when comparing patients who underwent PFO closure with control subjects. (*A*) Mean Reduction of Monthly Migraine Days, (*B*) Mean reduction of Monthly Migraine Attacks, (*C*) Responder Rate (%), (*D*) complete Cessation of Migraine. (Mohammad K. Mojadidi et al., Pooled Analysis of PFO Occluder Device Trials in Patients With PFO and Migraine, Journal of the American College of Cardiology, 77 (6), 2021, 667-676, https://doi.org/10.1016/j.jacc.2020.11.068.)

moderate to large right-to-left shunts and those who had failed multiple conventional therapies. It is unclear if these criteria enriched the trial cohorts with patients more likely to respond. However, they certainly made enrollment of the studies more difficult.

Based on this experience, if the true pathophysiologic relationship between PFO and migraine is ever to be understood and a randomized trial is ever going to prove a benefit of PFO closure for MHA sufferers, it will be critical that any future trial contains inclusion criteria which enable the investigators to select only the "causal" PFOs.

PLATELETS AND MIGRAINE HEADACHES

For decades, a platelet-mediated migraine mechanism has been suggested. Sicuteri and colleagues[36] demonstrated differences in metabolism of whole blood serotonin (a vasoconstrictor) in MHA sufferers compared with that of controls. Since virtually all the serotonin in whole blood is stored in the platelets, a primary platelet abnormality was suggested

by the authors as a migraine mechanism. Hilton and Cumings[37] demonstrated increased platelet aggregation (leading to serotonin release) in migraineurs compared with non-migraine controls. Deshmukh and Meyer[38] elegantly furthered the work of Sicuteri, by showing an increase in serum serotonin levels during the migraine prodrome with decreased levels during the headache phase.

The early use of platelet antagonists such as heparin, hirudin, methysergide, imipramine, dihydroergotamine, phentolamine, amitriptyline, aspirin, and phenylbutazone, for atherosclerosis and other clotting disorders, were anecdotally reported to produce secondary benefit on MHA frequency and severity.[39] As antiplatelet therapy became more sophisticated and more specific, there were a few case reports that ticlopidine, a platelet P2Y12-specific receptor inhibitor, also ameliorated headache symptoms.[40] Dipyridamole, another P2Y12 receptor inhibitor, was tested in a small series[41] but abandoned by the investigators when it actually worsened headache symptoms, due to its vasodilator effect, as was seen frequently in patients treated with coronary artery disease and stroke. Other investigators noted that smaller doses of dipyridamole had beneficial migraine effects without evidence of the vasodilator effect.[42,43]

Concurrent with the failed early Migraine–PFO trials, a number of authors reported de novo MHAs after transcatheter closure of atrial septal defects,[44–47] presumed to be related to platelet activation/aggregation on the surface of the implant. Several others reported the benefit of using ticlopidine[48,49] or clopidogrel[50,51] after the procedure to ameliorate these symptoms. Subsequently, Rodes-Cabau and a Canadian consortium published the CANOA Randomized Clinical Trial[52] in which patients undergoing transcatheter atrial septal defect (ASD) closure, with no prior history of migraines, were randomized to postimplant therapy, receiving either aspirin and clopidogrel or aspirin and a placebo. In the first 3 months after the procedure, patients in the dual antiplatelet cohort had fewer monthly migraine days, a lower incidence of migraine attacks, and less severe migraine attacks. The results suggested platelet activation/aggregation on the closure device's surface as a specific trigger for migraine in a subset of these patients.

In a study published in 2014, Chambers and colleagues[53] randomly assigned 80 episodic migraineurs (with and without PFO) to treatment with either clopidogrel or placebo. The study, which failed to fully enroll, showed no statistical difference in MHA reduction between the 2 treatment groups.

At the same time, Sommer and Robbins at Columbia University[54] first noted an unexpected reduction/elimination of migraine symptoms using clopidogrel to treat patients with prior stroke and PFO. They speculated that if platelet inhibition was successful in reducing the headache burden that there must be platelet aggregation or platelet activation by-products crossing the PFO from the systemic venous circulation to reach the brain in supraphysiologic levels, triggering the migraine symptoms. In a subsequent open-label observational series published in 2018,[55] they demonstrated a striking migraine reduction in 136 non-stroke migraineurs with PFO who had an average migraine burden of 14.8 days/month. While the impact of their results were limited by the use of unblinded/uncontrolled therapy, the authors demonstrated that successful platelet P2Y12 receptor inhibition with clopidogrel reduced MHA frequency by at least 50% in two-thirds of subjects tested (clopidogrel responders). There was a 57% clopidogrel responder rate in patients with episodic migraines, 61% in chronic migraineurs, 58% in patients with aura, 59% in patients without aura, 59% in patients with a small right to left (R to L) shunt, and 73% in patients with a moderate or large R to L shunt (all $P = NS$).

In the same cohort, using the commercially available, clinically validated VerifyNow Assay (Accriva Diagnostics, San Diego, CA), 16 of 17 clopidogrel responders had a PRU assay result less than 140, which was chosen to represent the minimally adequate platelet P2Y12 receptor inhibition for migraine effect (**Fig. 6**). Subsequently 45 of 56 clopidogrel nonresponders (<50% migraine frequency reduction) underwent PRU testing. Twenty-six of 45 had PRU levels less than 140. These 26 patients were considered to have been successfully platelet inhibited and were assumed to have an alternate (non-platelet, non-PFO) migraine mechanism.

The remaining 19 patients with PRU greater than 140 were considered inadequately platelet inhibited by clopidogrel. Sixteen of 19 were started on prasugrel, another P2Y12 specific thienopyridine with a different metabolic pathway than clopidogrel. On prasugrel, all 16 had a PRU value less

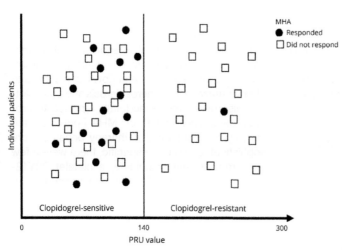

MHA
● Responded
☐ Did not respond

Clopidogrel-sensitive　　Clopidogrel-resistant

Individual patients

0　　　　140　　　　300
PRU value

Fig. 6. Clopidogrel MHA responders (*black circles*) are grouped below a PRU level of 140 with 1 outlier. Clopidogrel MHA nonresponders (*white squares*) fell into 2 groups: those below the criterion value of 140 considered adequately platelet inhibited and those above 140 who were inadequately platelet inhibited and who were subsequently treated with prasugrel. (Sommer, R. J., Nazif, T., Privitera, L., & Robbins, B. T. (2018). Retrospective review of thienopyridine therapy in migraineurs with patent foramen ovale. Neurology, 91(22), 1002–1009. https://doi.org/10.1212/wnl.0000000000006572.)

than 100. Six of 16 had no benefit in migraine symptoms (nonresponders) and were assumed to have a non-PFO migraine mechanism. The other 10 had greater than 50% migraine frequency reduction and met the same criteria for responder as those treated with clopidogrel. Overall, in this registry, 66% of the population responded to successful platelet P2Y12 receptor inhibition with 1 of the 2 thienopyridines.

With the assumption that a platelet by-product was crossing the PFO and triggering the headaches, 55 of the 90 thienopyridine responders (80 to clopidogrel, 10 to prasugrel) underwent subsequent off-label PFO closure with either the HELEX Septal Occluder or with the Cardioform Septal Occluder (W.L. Gore & Associates, Flagstaff, AZ) and were available for moderate-term follow-up. After discontinuation of the thienopyridine (3 months after implant), 52 of the 55 (94%) had ongoing effective migraine reduction, with a follow-up range to 6 years. All 8 thienopyridine responders who stopped P2Y12 inhibition without PFO closure had return of migraine symptoms at baseline levels within 4 to 5 days, the expected washout period for the medications. The duration of thienopyridine therapy did not change the observed return to baseline migraine activity. Based on the close correlation of response to thienopyridine and to closure, the authors speculated that thienopyridine responsiveness could be used as a test to identify the migraine patients with "causal" PFOs for clinical practice and for future migraine-PFO trials.

In a concurrent investigator-initiated cohort of 40 migraine–PFO patients,[56] the Columbia group also demonstrated clinical migraine benefit (>50% monthly headache reduction) with ticagrelor, a non-thienopyridine platelet P2Y12 receptor specific inhibitor. The medication has a similar mechanism of action to dipyridamole, causing increased levels of extracellular adenosine, which is both a vasodilator stimulus and major mediator of inflammation. Like with the use of dipyridamole in this population, in the ticagrelor-migraine study, a number of subjects had a transient initial increase in headaches and a variety of other systemic symptoms not seen with the thienopyridines.

In 2021, Trabbatoni and Camera[57] in a remarkable benchtop series, demonstrated a unique platelet hyperactivity in patients with migraine and PFO. Using advanced cell sorting techniques including flow cytometry and mass spectrometry, the authors showed a markedly increased platelet thrombin-generating capacity, characterized by the expression of tissue factor on the cell surface of platelets and platelet-derived microvesicles. At the same time, the patients seemed to have an altered oxidative stress state, with increased platelet reactive oxidative species, and an increased ratio of oxidized to reduced glutathione. Return to normal platelet physiology and a normal oxidative stress state was demonstrated 6 months after PFO closure. In a separate analysis, after treatment of the blood in vitro with clopidogrel metabolites, platelet status and oxidative stress state returned to normal (statistically similar to control subjects with neither migraine nor PFO).

THE GORE RELIEF CLINICAL STUDY

The GORE RELIEF Clinical Study (clinicaltrials.gov; Study Number: NCT04100135)[58,59] was designed collaboratively by a working group of interventional cardiologists, headache neurologists, and regulators from the FDA based on the concept that thienopyridines could be used as a screening tool for identifying the causal PFO. It is a randomized, double-blinded, placebo and sham-controlled trial. The trial is currently enrolling in the United States.

Migraineurs with more than 1 headache day per week (chronic migraine and high-frequency episodic migraine), who meet ICHA 3 guidelines for migraine with or without aura, and who have failed at least 2 classes of established migraine preventative therapy will be considered for enrollment in RELIEF. Those who meet the entrance criteria will be screened for a right-to-left shunt using either transcranial Doppler, transthoracic echo, or transesophageal echo with intravenous agitated saline injection (both with and without Valsalva). Those subjects with at least a moderate R to L shunt will be enrolled and will keep an electronic headache log to establish a baseline headache frequency. Those with a sufficient number of migraine days during this tracking period will continue to the medication/enrichment phase of the trial.

All study medications will be over-encapsulated, allowing for effective blinding of the subjects. Most subjects will be loaded with and started on clopidogrel 75 mg daily. A small cohort will be loaded with a matching placebo tablet and will take placebo daily, to establish a control group to assess the efficacy of the thienopyridine. After 1 week, subjects will undergo PRU testing to determine adequate platelet inhibition. Those taking clopidogrel with a PRU less than 140 will remain on daily clopidogrel. Those taking clopidogrel with a PRU greater than 140 will be switched to matching over-encapsulated prasugrel, maintaining the blind. Those on placebo will remain on daily placebo. The number of migraine days on medication will then be compared with the number of migraine days at baseline. Only the thienopyridine-treated patients with a $\geq$ 50% reduction in headache frequency (responders) will continue to the catheterization laboratory phase of the trial.

In the catheterization laboratory, femoral venous access will be obtained as for any other PFO closure case. After assessing right heart pressures, a wire will be advanced across the PFO as a final study entrance criterion. Then, under deep conscious sedation with sensory deprivation (blindfold, headphones), the patients will be randomized 1:1 to PFO closure with the GORE Cardioform Septal Occluder (W.L. Gore & Associates, Flagstaff AZ; **Fig. 7**), or to a sham procedure in which the sheaths and catheters will simply be removed. Blinding of the patient to procedural outcomes, blinding of the staff caring for the patient, and blinding of the study neurologist will be maintained.

The patient will remain on open-label thienopyridine for the next 4 months. The drug will then be stopped, and headache monitoring will be resumed. The primary efficacy end point of the trial will be the comparison of the reduction of headache frequency (days/month) after discontinuation of thienopyridine in the closure group versus the sham group. Patients in the trial who were randomized to the sham cohort will be eligible for closure at the completion of the trial should they so desire.

The goal of the GORE RELIEF Clinical Study is to use thienopyridine responsiveness to select only patients with causal PFO. To maximize enrollment, and to assess the impact of the therapy on the largest group of migraineurs possible, the trial allows for a wide range of migraine patients, permitting both chronic and episodic migraine patients as well as those with and without migraine aura. The assumption of the trial designers is that the patients with a positive response to the blinded thienopyridine therapy will select themselves for the randomized catheter treatment. Two of the other trial-specific selection criteria were chosen for reasons having little to do with enriching the study cohort. The requirement of a moderate or large right-to-left shunt was chosen to make sure that the PFO could be identified and crossed during the catheterization laboratory procedure. The requirement that patients had failed at least 2 preventive therapies from different classes of medication was chosen to exclude patients who had not previously undergone tests of established therapy prior to the use of an invasive/experimental procedure.

SUMMARY

With our current limited understanding of migraine pathophysiology, we are far from a future in which baseline testing will determine the optimal medication or combination of medications for each patient. Today, the selection of medication for every patient is undertaken entirely on a trial-and-error basis. While the available medical therapies fall into many drug classes, many have untenable side effects and extreme financial costs which lead to frequent discontinuation and all have the need for lifelong treatment. Once stopped, the migraine symptoms will return.

The role of PFO in migraine patients remains controversial and unproven. Most experts agree that there is an association between PFO and migraine, but there is little consensus on how the two are linked physiologically. A platelet-mediated mechanism seems to be present in some patients, and for that subset of migraine sufferers platelet P2Y12 receptor inhibition may potentially offer a new alternative class of therapy. The RELIEF Study is not designed to explain the physiology of the P2Y12/platelet connection to migraine. But if it is a successful trial, it should not only lead to more focused basic science investigation, but also could provide an alternative of a low-risk, one-time procedure instead of lifelong medication, which would likely be of great interest to many patients.

While the RELIEF cohort of high-frequency episodic or chronic migraines is a simple population in whom to test the effect of antiplatelet therapy, the use of thienopyridines would be impractical for many other migraine patient groups. For example, it would be much more difficult, and take far longer, to adequately assess the thienopyridine response of patients with severe but infrequent migraines, or of

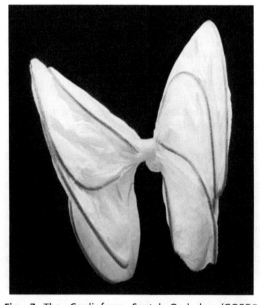

Fig. 7. The Cardioform Septal Occluder (GORE® HELEX® Septal Occluder and GORE® CARDIOFORM Septal Occluder. See Instructions for Use for complete device information, including approved indications and safety information.).

patients with clustered migraine attacks. For these patients, the hope is that novel laboratory platelet testing strategies will lead to a "migraine panel" of blood tests which could determine PFO causality. Having such an objective set of data would eliminate the need for the blood thinner trials, their associated bleeding/bruising risks and any placebo effect which might be associated with their use.

At a minimum, a successful outcome of the RELIEF Clinical Study will require a change in the paradigm for neurologic evaluation of migraineurs to include screening for a right-to-left shunt and a trial of antiplatelet therapy. If the patient responds positively to antiplatelet medication, whether the patient then chooses chronic antiplatelet therapy or a PFO closure would be a personal decision to be made with their treating physician. But the critical first step is to excite the migraine neurology community and the patients themselves, about the possibilities of the RELIEF Clinical Study. Completing RELIEF represents the best opportunity to date, to prove a benefit of PFO closure in a subset of migraineurs.

CLINICS CARE POINTS

- The underlying pathophysiology of migraine headaches remains poorly understood.

- There are scant evidence-based data to support the use of patent foramen ovale (PFO) closure as a migraine therapy. As such, it is not approved for this indication in the United States.

- The failure of the early migraine–PFO closure trials was based in part on the inability to select patients in whom the PFO was mechanistically related ("causal") to the migraine symptoms, from those in whom the PFO was an incidental finding.

- A critical mass of observational and basic research data suggests a platelet-mediated mechanism in a subset of migraine patients.

- The GORE RELIEF Clinical Study, a study designed to select only the causal PFOs, using thienopyridine responsiveness as an inclusion criterion, is currently enrolling and has the best chance to prove the benefit of PFO closure in a subset of migraine patients.

DISCLOSURE

R. Sommer is the National Cardiology Principal Investigator for the GORE RELIEF Clinical Study. Columbia University receives institutional support for Dr R. Sommer's work on the trial from the sponsor W.L. Gore & Associates.

REFERENCES

1. Safiri S, Pourfathi H, Eagan A, et al. Global, regional, and national burden of migraine in 204 countries and territories, 1990 to 2019. Pain 2022;163(2):e293–309.
2. GBD 2019 Diseases and Injuries Collaborators. Global burden of 369 diseases and injuries in 204 countries and territories, 1990–2019: a systematic analysis for the Global Burden of Disease Study 2019. Lancet 2020;396:1204–22.
3. Clifford Rose F. The history of migraine from Mesopotamian to medieval times. Cephalalgia 1995;(Suppl 15):1–3.
4. Rabkin R, Stables D, Levin N, et al. The prophylactic value of propranolol in angina pectoris. Am J Cardiol 1966;18:370–83.
5. Pelzer N, Stam AH, Haan J, et al. Familial and sporadic hemiplegic migraine: diagnosis and treatment. Curr Treat Options Neurol 2013;15(1):13–27.
6. Brin MF, Swope DM, O'Brian C, et al. Botox for migraine: double-bind, placebo-controlled region-specific evaluation. Cephalalgia 2000;20:421–2.
7. Silberstein S, Mathew N, Saper J, et al. Botulinum toxin type A as a migraine preventive treatment. For the BOTOX Migraine Clinical Research Group. Headache 2000;40:445–50.
8. Chronicle EP, Mulleners WM. Anticonvulsant drugs for migraine prophylaxis. Cochrane Database Syst Rev 2004;3.
9. Tronvik E, Stovner LJ, Helde G, et al. Prophylactic treatment of migraine with an angiotensin II receptor blocker: a randomized controlled trial. JAMA 2003; 289:65–9.
10. Punay NC, Couch JR. Antidepressants in the treatment of migraine headache. Curr Pain Headache Rep 2003;7:51–4.
11. Arca K, Reynolds J, Sands KA, et al. Calcitonin gene-related peptide antagonists for the prevention of migraine: highlights from pivotal studies and the clinical relevance of this new drug class. Ann Pharmacother 2020 Aug;54(8):795–803.
12. Burstein R, Noseda R, Borsook D. Migraine: multiple Processes, complex pathophysiology. J Neuroscience 2015;35:6619–29.
13. Tzourio C, Tehindrazanarivelo A, Iglesias S, et al. Case-control study of migraine and risk of ischaemic stroke in young women. BMJ 1995;310:830–3.
14. Henrich JB, Horwitz RI. A controlled study of ischemic stroke risk in migraine patients. J Clin Epidemiol 1989;42(8):773–80.
15. Lechat P, Mas JL, Lascault G, et al. Prevalence of patent foramen ovale in patients with stroke. NEJM 1988;318:1148–52.

16. Webster MWI, Smith HJ, Sharpe DN, et al. Patent foramen ovale in young stroke patients. Lancet 1988; 2:11–2.

17. Anzola GP, Magoni M, Guindani M, et al. Potential source of cerebral embolism in migraine with aura: a transcranial Doppler study. Neurology 1999;52: 1622–5.

18. Schwedt TJ, Demaerschalk BM, Dodick DW. Patent foramen ovale and migraine: a quantitative systematic review. Cephalalgia 2008;28:531–40.

19. Truong T, Slavin L, Kashani R, et al. Prevalence of migraine headache in patients with congenital heart disease. Am J Cardiol 2008;101:396–400.

20. Post MC, van Gent MWF, Plokker HWM, et al. Pulmonary arteriovenous malformations associated with migraine with aura. Eur Respir J 2009;34:882–7.

21. Wilmshurst PT, Nightingale S, Walsh KP, et al. Effect on migraine of closure of cardiac right-to-left shunts to prevent recurrence of decompression illness or stroke or for haemodynamic reasons. Lancet 2000; 356:1648–51.

22. Morandi E, Anzola GP, Angeli S, et al. Transcatheter closure of patent foramen ovale: a new migraine treatment? J Int Cardiol 2003;16:39–42.

23. Schwerzmann M, Wiher S, Nedeltchev K, et al. Percutaneous closure of patent foramen ovale reduces the frequency of migraine attacks. Neurology 2004;62:1399–401.

24. Giardini A, Donti A, Formigari R, et al. Transcatheter patent foramen ovale closure mitigates aura migraine headaches abolishing spontaneous right-to-left shunting. Am Heart J 2006;151:922.e1–5.

25. Reisman M, Christofferson RD, Jesurum J, et al. Migraine headache relief after transcatheter closure of patent foramen ovale. J Am Coll Cardiol 2005;45: 493–5.

26. Slavin L, Tobis JM, Rangarajan K, et al. Five-year experience with percutaneous closure of patent foramen ovale. Am J Cardiol 2007;99:1316–20.

27. Kimmelstiel C, Gange C, Thaler D. Is patent foramen ovale closure effective in reducing migraine symptoms? A controlled study. Catheter Cardiovasc Interv 2007;69:740–6.

28. Papa M, Gaspardone A, Fragasso G, et al. Usefulness of transcatheter patent foramen ovale closure in migraineurs with moderate to large right-to-left shunt and instrumental evidence of cerebrovascular damage. Am J Cardiol 2009;104:434–9.

29. Wahl A, Praz F, Tai T, et al. Improvement of migraine headaches after percutaneous closure of patent foramen ovale for secondary prevention of paradoxical embolism. Heart 2010;96(12):967–73.

30. Khessali H, Mojadidi MK, Gevorgyan R, et al. The effect of patent foramen ovale closure on visual aura without headache or typical aura with migraine headache. JACC Cardiovasc Interv 2012;5(6): 682–7.

31. Dowson A, Mullen MJ, Peatfield R, et al. Migraine Intervention with STARFlex Technology (MIST) trial: a prospective, multicenter, double-blind, sham-controlled trial to evaluate the effectiveness of patent foramen ovale closure with STARFlex septal repair implant to resolve refractory migraine headache. Circulation 2008;117:1397–404.

32. ESCAPE migraine trial. Available at: https://clinicaltrials. gov/study/NCT00267371?cond=Migraine%20Head ache&term=Patent%20Foramen%20Ovale&page=2 &rank=15.

33. Mattle HP, Evers S, Hildick-Smith D, et al. Percutaneous closure of patent foramen ovale in migraine with aura: a randomized controlled trial. Eur Heart J 2016;37(26):2029–36.

34. Tobis JM, Charles A, Silberstein SD, et al. Percutaneous closure of patent foramen ovale in patients with migraine: the PREMIUM Trial. J Am Coll Cardiol 2017;70:2766–74.

35. Mojadidi MK, Kumar P, Mahmoud AN, et al. Pooled analysis of PFO occluder device trials in patients with PFO and migraine. J Am Coll Cardiol 2021;77:667–76.

36. Sicuteri F, Testi A, Anselmi B. Biochemical investigations in headache: increase in Hydroxyindoleactic Acid Excretion during migraine attacks. Int Arch Allergy Appl Immun 1961;19:55.

37. Hilton BP, Cumings JN. 5-Hydroxytryptamine levels and platelet aggregation responses in subjects with acute migraine headache. J Neurology, Neurosurgery, and Psychiatry 1972;35:505–9.

38. Deshmukh SV, Meyer JS. Cyclic changes in platelet dynamics and the pathogenesis and prophylaxis of migraine. Headache 1977;17:101–8.

39. Hanington E. Migraine: a blood disorder? Lancet 1978;2:501–3.

40. Bousser MG, Conard J, Lecrubier C, et al. Migraine or transient ischemic attacks in a patient with essential thrombocythaemia. Treatment with ticlopidine. Ann Med Interne 1980;131(2):87–90.

41. Hawkes CH. Dipyridamole in migraine. Lancet 1978; 2:153.

42. Dalessio DJ. Use of platelet antagonists in the treatment of migraine. Headache 1976;16:129–30.

43. Damasio H. Success of failure of dipyridamole in migraine. Lancet 1978;2:478–9.

44. Rodes-Cabau J, Molina C, Serrano-Munuera C, et al. Migraine with aura related to the percutaneous closure of an atrial septal defect. Catheter Cardiovasc Interv 2003;60:540–2.

45. Fernandez-Mayoralas DM, Fernandez-Jaen A, Munoz-Jareno N, et al. Migraine symptoms related to the percutaneous closure of an ostium secundum atrial septal defect: report of four paediatric cases and review of the literature. Cephalalgia 2007;27:550–6.

46. Mortelmans K, Post M, Thijs V, et al. The influence of percutaneous atrial septal defect closure on the occurrence of migraine. Eur Heart J 2005;26:1533–7.

47. Yew G, Wilson NJ. Transcatheter atrial septal defect closure with the Amplatzer septal occluder: five-year follow-up. Catheter Cardiovasc Interv 2005;64: 193–6.

48. Tomita H, Hatakeyama K, Soda W, et al. Efficacy of ticlopidine for preventing migraine after transcatheter closure of atrial septal defect with Amplatzer septal occluder: a case report. J Cardiol 2007;49: 357–60.

49. Benemei S, Rossi E, Marcucci R, et al. Atrial septal defect closure and de novo migraine: exclusive ticlopidine efficacy. Cephalalgia 2012 Nov;32(15): 1144–6.

50. Sharifi M, Burks J. Efficacy of clopidogrel in the treatment of post-ASD closure migraines. Catheter Cardiovasc Interv 2004;63:255.

51. Wilmshurst PT, Nightingale S, Walsh KP, et al. Clopidogrel reduces migraine with aura after transcatheter closure of persistent foramen ovale and atrial septal defects. Heart 2005;91:1173–5.

52. Rodes-Cabau J, Horlick E, Ibrahim R, et al. Effect of clopidogrel and aspirin vs aspirin alone on migraine headaches after transcatheter atrial septal defect closure: the CANOA Randomized Clinical Trial. JAMA 2015;314:2147–54.

53. Chambers JB, Seed PT, Ridsdale L. Clopidogrel as prophylactic treatment for migraine: a pilot randomised, controlled study. Cephalalgia 2014;34: 1163–8.

54. Spencer BT, Qureshi Y, Sommer RJ. A retrospective review of clopidogrel as primary therapy for migraineurs with right to left shunt lesions. Cephalalgia 2014;34:933–7.

55. Sommer RJ, Nazif T, Privitera L, et al. Retrospective review of thienopyridine therapy in migraineurs with patent foramen ovale. Neurology 2018;91:1002–9.

56. Reisman AM, Robbins BT, Chou DE, et al. Ticagrelor for refractory migraine/patent foramen ovale (TRACTOR): an open-label pilot study. Neurology 2018;91:1010–7.

57. Trabattoni D, Brambilla M, Canzano P, et al. Migraine in patients undergoing PFO closure: characterization of a platelet-associated pathophysiological mechanism: the LEARNER Study. J Am Coll Cardiol Basic Transl Sci 2022;7:525–40.

58. The GORE RELIEF clinical study. Available at: https://clinicaltrials.gov/study/NCT04100135.

59. The GORE RELIEF clinical study. Available at: www.reliefclinicalstudy.com.

Patent Foramen Ovale and Hypoxemia

Ashley Nguyen, DO[a], Elaine Nguyen, MD[b], Preetham Kumar, MD[c],*

KEYWORDS

- Chronic bronchitis • Chronic obstructive pulmonary disease • Emphysema
- Obstructive sleep apnea • Patent foramen ovale • Platypnea-orthodeoxia syndrome

KEY POINTS

- Although patent foramen ovale has commonly been associated with cryptogenic stroke and migraines, it has also been shown to be linked with a few hypoxemic conditions, such platypnea orthodeoxia syndrome, obstructive sleep apnea, and chronic obstructive pulmonary disease, out of proportion to the severity of the underlying pulmonary disease.
- The evidence supporting this link is not as strong as that for patent foramen ovale and cryptogenic stroke and migraines, so there are no guidelines for the diagnosis and management of the interatrial shunt in such conditions.
- Despite the lack of consensus statements regarding patent foramen ovale and the aforementioned hypoxemic conditions from major medical associations, the health care team, in the appropriate setting, should include it in its differential to ensure optimal patient care.

PART 1: PLATYPNEA-ORTHODEOXIA SYNDROME

Introduction

Platypnea-orthodeoxia syndrome (POS), first described by Burchell and colleagues[1] in 1949, is a rare condition characterized by dyspnea and hypoxemia when switching from a supine position to an upright or standing position. Objectively, orthodeoxia is defined by a drop in arterial oxygen tension (Pao_2) by greater than 4 mm Hg or arterial oxyhemoglobin saturation (SaO2) by greater than 5% greater than when switching from the supine position to the upright position.

Prevalence

To date, less than 200 case reports and series exist describing POS, and approximately 100 case reports and series exist describing POS in the setting of PFO, highlighting the rarity of this clinical syndrome. Since the diagnosis of POS is often not considered in the differential diagnosis of hypoxemia, it is likely that the condition is underreported.

Pathophysiology

The pathophysiology of POS is not fully understood yet, but it appears to require an anatomic component and a functional component, and these 2 components produce right-to-left shunting of deoxygenated blood.

The anatomic component enables direct communication between the deoxygenated venous system and oxygenated arterial system. Examples of an anatomic component include an intracardiac shunt, such as a patent foramen ovale (PFO) or atrial septal defect, and intrapulmonary shunt, such as pulmonary arteriovenous malformation and ventilation-perfusion mismatch.

The functional component increases the pressure gradient at the atrial level between the venous and arterial systems such that the venous system drains into the arterial system. Examples of a

a Department of Medicine, Cleveland Clinic Florida, 2950 Cleveland Clinic Boulevard, Weston, FL 33331, USA; b Division of Pulmonary and Critical Care Medicine, Department of Medicine, Riverside University Health System, 26520 Cactus Avenue, Moreno Valley, CA 92555, USA; c Division of Cardiology, Department of Medicine, University of California, Riverside, 900 University Avenue, Riverside, CA 92521, USA
* Corresponding author.
E-mail address: pk.kumarp.316@gmail.com

Cardiol Clin 42 (2024) 509–519
https://doi.org/10.1016/j.ccl.2024.01.008

functional component can be broken down into 2 groups of conditions: one that alters cardiac anatomy to redirect blood entering the right atrium toward the interatrial communication instead of the right ventricle (eg, aortic root dilatation, atrial septal aneurysm, prominent Eustachian valve) and another that reverses the pressure gradient between the 2 atria (eg, chronic obstructive pulmonary disease [COPD] and pulmonary hypertension).

Table 1 summarizes a list of conditions that have been reported to be associated with POS.

Diagnosis and Evaluation

Since diagnosis of POS requires documentation of significant oxygen desaturation upon assuming an upright posture, evaluation can include pulse oximetry, arterial blood gas, or right heart catheterization.

Treatment and Outcomes

Multiple case reports and case series exist describing the evaluation and management of POS secondary to PFO.[2–5]

One common presentation is of a patient who develops hypoxemia following surgery in which the degree of oxygen desaturation is out of proportion to the degree of pre-existing pulmonary disease. Since physicians are usually unaware that patients in their practice have a PFO, several weeks might pass before someone thinks about right-to-left shunting through a PFO as a cause of the hypoxemia.

Table 1
Mechanism of platypnea-orthodeoxia syndrome

Intracardiac Shunt	
Normal Right Atrial Pressure + Preferential Blood Flow Across the Interatrial Defect due to an Intracardiac Anatomic Defect	Aortic valve replacement/repair[11] Ascending aortic aneurysm/elongation/ tortuosity[12–18] Atrial thrombus[19] Cardiac mass[20] Eosinophilic endomyocardial disease[21] Lipomatous hypertrophy of interatrial septum[22] Persistent left superior vena cava[23] Prominent Eustachian valve[24] Tricuspid regurgitation/stenosis[25]
Normal Right Atrial Pressure + Preferential Blood Flow Across the Interatrial Defect Due to an Extracardiac Anatomic Defect	Blunt chest trauma[25,26] Hemidiaphragm paralysis[27] Hepatic Hydatid cyst (large)[28] Kyphosis (severe)[29] Paraesophageal hernia[30]
Elevated Right Atrial Pressure OR Transient Reversal of Left-to-Right Atrial Pressure Gradient	Constrictive pericarditis[31,32] Pericardial effusion[33] Pneumonectomy[34] Pulmonary embolism[35]
Extracardiac Shunt	
Intrapulmonary shunt	Acute respiratory distress syndrome[36] Hepato-pulmonary syndrome[37]
Ventilation-perfusion mismatch	Cryptogenic organizing fibrosis[38] Interstitial lung disease[39] Pneumonectomy[40–42]
Miscellaneous	
Amiodarone lung toxicity[43]	
Bronchogenic carcinoma[44]	
Diabetic autonomic neuropathy[45]	
Fat embolism[46]	
Ileus[47]	
Organophosphorus poisoning[48]	
Parkinson's disease[49]	
Radiation-induced bronchial stenosis[50]	
Traumatic bronchial rupture[51]	

Kamel and colleagues[2] describe a 54-year-old man with POS due to net right-to-left shunting through a PFO in the setting of metastatic cholangiosarcoma associated with extracardiac lymphadenopathy compressing the right atrium, thereby increasing the pressure in this chamber, whose symptoms improved following successful PFO closure. His resting peripheral oxygen saturation increased from 90% on 6 L per minute from nasal cannula to 100% on room air.

Similarly, Sitbon and colleagues[3] describe an 87-year-old woman with POS due to net right-to-left shunting through a PFO secondary to a dilated thoracic aorta compressing the right atrium as shown by 4-dimensional flow MRI, whose dyspnea and hypoxemia improved following PFO closure.

Mojadidi and colleagues[6] performed a single-center prospective study looking at change in SaO_2 before and after PFO closure in patients with POS. Among 17 such individuals, 11/17 (64.8%) experienced an improvement in recumbent SaO_2 (90.5 ± 6.9% pre-closure vs 95.7 ± 2.1% post-closure, $P = .03$) and standing SaO_2 (76.3 ± 5.2% pre-closure vs 91.7 ± 7.8% post-closure, $P<.0001$). The remaining 6 patients who did not experience a similar relief had pulmonary hypertension with a mean pulmonary artery pressure (PAP) of 50 mm Hg, leading to the belief that the hypoxemia in this subgroup was predominantly due to a pulmonary issue.

Shah and colleagues describe a single-center series involving 52 patients with POS associated with a PFO who underwent transcatheter closure of PFO, either with a dedicated PFO device or non-PFO device, and all the patients demonstrated immediate improvements in oxygen saturations.[7]

Similarly, Blanche and colleagues describe a single-center series involving 5 patients with POS associated with a PFO who underwent percutaneous PFO closure, and all the patients showed immediate improvements in mean arterial oxygen saturations in the upright position (83% ± 3% to 93% ± 2%) with complete resolution of symptoms.[8]

Fig. 1 and Video 1 illustrate a 70-year-old female with a history of migraines since her teenage years, right hemidiaphragm paralysis, POS, and PFO complaining of dyspnea associated with hypoxemia when assuming an upright position who experienced relief in symptoms associated with her POS following PFO closure with a 35 mm Cribriform Amplatzer Occluder device. During initial evaluation, an inferior vena cava venogram was performed, and it showed a torrent of blood flow from the right atrium into the left atrium. Following PFO closure, a repeat inferior vena cava venogram

was performed, and it showed no blood flow to the left atrium through the PFO. This resulted in complete cessation of the dyspnea, hypoxemia, and migraines.

Fig. 2 shows the transesophageal echocardiogram of an 85-year-old male with a history of stroke complicated by profound hypoxemia associated with loss of independence. His oxygen saturation on room air was 96% while lying flat, and it fell to the low 70s while standing upright. He continued to experience severe dyspnea despite being on 6 L per minute of nasal oxygen. After spending over a week in the hospital for further evaluation and management of the severe hypoxemia, his physicians considered PFO as a possible culprit. Consequently, the PFO was closed with a 30 mm Gore Cardioform Septal Occluder. His oxygen saturation on room air improved from low 70s to 94% while standing upright, and his dyspnea resolved. The patient was safely discharged home the following day so that he could resume his independent lifestyle.

Summary

Given the low prevalence of POS associated with a PFO, it would be challenging to conduct a randomized controlled trial (RCT) assessing the safety and efficacy of percutaneous PFO closure in patients with POS due to PFO. However, an impressive amount of observational evidence exists in the scientific literature that shows complete resolution of POS upon PFO closure. Accordingly, without randomized clinical trials, the 2021 European Society of Cardiology guidelines give a "strong" recommendation and 2022 Society for Cardiovascular Angiography and Interventions guidelines give a "conditional" recommendation for PFO closure in this patient population.[9,10] Consequently, clinicians should be vigilant about assessing for POS in any patient presenting with dyspnea and hypoxemia out of proportion to the degree of pulmonary disease. In this setting, one should consider PFO with extensive right-to-left shunting of deoxygenated blood as the mechanistic etiology. Furthermore, a PFO with this high degree of right-to-left shunting represents a form of cyanotic congenital heart disease, and percutaneous PFO closure is the appropriate treatment.

PART 2: OBSTRUCTIVE SLEEP APNEA
Introduction

Obstructive sleep apnea (OSA), the most common sleep-related breathing disorder, is a condition characterized by episodes of apnea and hypopnea secondary to collapse of the upper airway. Risk factors for OSA include older age, male sex,

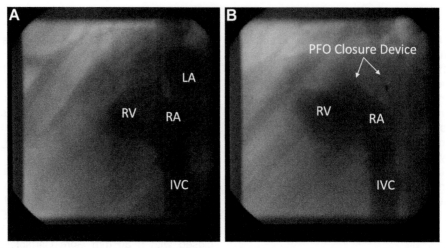

Fig. 1. (*A*) IVC angiogram of a 70-year-old female with POS and PFO who experienced relief related to POS following (*B*) PFO closure with a 35-mm Cribriform Amplatzer Occluder device. IVC, inferior vena cava; LA, left atrium; PFO, patent foramen ovale; POS, platypnea-orthodeoxia syndrome; RA, right atrium; RV, right ventricle.

obesity, and anatomic (craniofacial and upper airway) abnormalities. Conditions commonly associated with OSA include obesity hypoventilation syndrome, congestive heart failure, atrial fibrillation, pulmonary hypertension, systemic hypertension, end-stage renal disease, chronic lung disease, stroke, and pregnancy. A less well-established condition associated with OSA is the presence of a PFO. This section will focus on OSA and PFO.

Prevalence of Patent Foramen Ovale in Obstructive Sleep Apnea

Based on large-scale epidemiology studies, the prevalence of OSA in North America is estimated to be approximately 15% to 30% in males and 10% to 15% in females.[52] On the other hand, the prevalence of PFO associated with OSA is less clear primarily due to a lack of data. Shanoudy and colleagues[53] assessed the prevalence of PFO in patients with OSA utilizing contrast transesophageal echocardiography (TEE), and they found that 33/48 (69%) OSA patients had a PFO, compared to 4/24 (17%) controls. Beelke and colleagues[54] conducted a similar study using transcranial Doppler (TCD), a diagnostic test with higher sensitivity for detecting PFO compared to TEE, and they found that 21/78 (27%) OSA patients, compared to 13/89 (15%) controls, had a PFO. Mojadidi and colleagues[55] assessed the presence of PFO, diagnosed using a TCD, in patients with OSA. The frequency of PFO in OSA

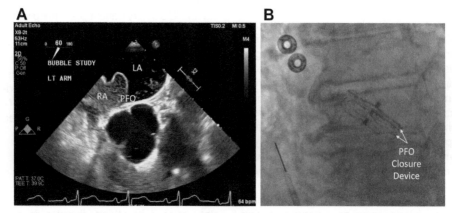

Fig. 2. An 85-year-old male with a history of POS whose (*A*) transesophageal echocardiogram with bubble study showed a PFO with hypermobile atrial septal aneurysm who experienced relief in dyspnea and hypoxemia following (*B*) PFO closure with a 30-mm Gore Cardioform Septal Occluder. LA, left atrium; PFO, patent foramen ovale; POS, platypnea-orthodeoxia syndrome; RA, right atrium.

was 2-fold greater than in control subjects without OSA. Furthermore, they found that 42% of the 100 OSA patients, compared to 19% of the 200 controls, had a PFO (P<.0001).

Hemodynamics of Obstructive Sleep Apnea Relevant to Patent Foramen Ovale

During an episode of apnea-hypopnea, the airway collapses, and the ongoing inspiratory effort against a fixed obstruction creates a vacuum in the chest cavity. The associated drop in intrathoracic pressure decreases preload, but when the patient inhales again, there is increased venous return to the right atrium, which can open the PFO, resulting in a right-to-left shunt. Johansson and colleagues[56] showed that OSA patients with PFO, compared to OSA patients without PFO, had a significantly higher proportion of oxygen desaturation to respiratory events (0.66 vs 0.33, P<.001). This implies that the presence of a PFO makes the symptoms associated with OSA appear earlier compared to subjects with OSA but without a PFO based on the observation that PFO exacerbates the oxygen desaturation inherently associated with apnea-hypopnea episodes. Further studies are needed to better elucidate the exact mechanism of the relationship between PFO and OSA.

Is Patent Foramen Ovale Responsible for Increasing Stroke Risk in Patients with Obstructive Sleep Apnea?

Numerous studies highlight an association between OSA and stroke. Loke and colleagues[57] pooled 9 prospective studies looking into OSA and stroke incidence, and they found that the presence of OSA increased the risk of developing a stroke (odds ratio [OR] = 2.24, 95% confidence interval [CI] 1.57–3.19, P<.001). Xie and colleagues pooled 16 cohort studies reporting the association between OSA of differing severities and stroke, and they found that severe OSA was associated with an increased risk of stroke (relative risk [RR] = 2.15, 95% CI 1.42–3.24, P<.001).[58] This relationship exists even after adjusting for confounding variables, such as age, sex, race, body mass index, presence of atrial fibrillation, smoking status, and alcohol consumption status, implying the presence of an independent yet undiscovered mechanism.

From a metabolic basis, OSA is associated with a prothrombotic state, placing patients at an increased risk for thrombus formation. Since many of these patients are obese, they have increased venous pressures which would predispose to stasis and venous thrombosis. In this setting of hypercoagulability, the coexistence of a PFO could provide the pathway for a paradoxic embolism. Future studies on the association of OSA and stroke need to assess the presence of PFO in this population.

Clinical Implications of Assessing and Closing Patent Foramen Ovale in Patients with Obstructive Sleep Apnea

Since OSA patients, compared to non-OSA patients, have a higher PFO prevalence and are at an increased risk for stroke, and PFO presence exacerbates the oxygen desaturation associated with the apnea-hypopnea episodes characteristic of OSA, it is reasonable to screen OSA patients for PFO. However, data regarding efficacy of PFO closure for stroke prevention and relief of symptoms related to OSA in OSA patients are lacking. Silver and colleagues[59] discuss a 51-year-old male with OSA whose frequency of apneas and hypopneas significantly decreased after PFO closure. Rimoldi and colleagues[60] report significant improvement in the apnea-hypopnea index, oxygen desaturation index, and OSA severity after PFO closure in OSA patients with PFO compared to OSA patients without PFO. Culpepper and colleagues[61] describe a 38-year-old male with severe OSA complicated by significant nocturnal hypoxemia despite compliance with a continuous positive airway pressure (CPAP) machine. The subject also had a PFO, which was closed percutaneously, and this led to complete resolution of nocturnal hypoxemia despite the persistence of OSA. Although a randomized clinical trial of PFO closure to reduce the symptoms and hypoxemia of OSA is feasible, an RCT has not been funded yet by the manufacturing companies.

PART 3: CHRONIC OBSTRUCTIVE PULMONARY DISEASE WITH HYPOXEMIA OUT OF PROPORTION TO PULMONARY DISEASE
Introduction

COPD is a preventable and treatable chronic lung disease that is marked by persistent, and often progressive, airflow obstruction that is not completely reversible due to varying degrees of airway inflammation (bronchitis/bronchiolitis) and/or alveolar destruction (emphysema).[62] Due to heterogeneity in clinical presentation, COPD is frequently misdiagnosed or underdiagnosed. Symptoms can vary, with the most common ones being chest tightness, chronic cough, dyspnea, sputum expectoration, and wheezing. The cause of COPD is multifactorial, including, but not limited to, environmental factors (eg, exposure to air pollution and tobacco smoke), recurrent or severe respiratory infections, genetics, and abnormal lung development. As per COPD guidelines, spirometry demonstrating a post-bronchodilator forced expiratory volume in 1 second (FEV_1)/forced vital capacity (FVC) of less than 0.7 is required to establish the diagnosis.[63]

Prevalence of Patent Foramen Ovale in Chronic Obstructive Pulmonary Disease

In 1999, Soliman and colleagues[64] were the first to compare the prevalence of PFO in patients with severe COPD (defined in the study as FEV_1/FVC<0.5 and FEV_1 < 50%) and controls. Using TEE with contrast, a PFO was identified in 14/20 (70%) patients with severe COPD and in 7/20 (35%) controls ($P<.05$). Similarly, Hacievliyagil and colleagues[65] noted that a PFO was detected in 23/52 (44%) COPD patients compared to 10/50 (20%) controls ($P<.01$). Lastly, Kilic and colleagues[66] observed a PFO prevalence of 4/21 (19%) in patients with mild COPD and Martolini and colleagues[67] observed a PFO prevalence of 12/22 (54%) in patients with moderate COPD.

In contrast, Shaik and colleagues[68], using both transthoracic echocardiogram and TCD, reported no significant difference in PFO prevalence between COPD and control groups (23/50 [46%] and 15/50 [30%], respectively, $P = .15$) irrespective of PFO shunt size or COPD severity. However, a sub-group analysis demonstrated a significantly greater prevalence of PFO with large shunt magnitude (defined as TCD grade 4–5) in patients with severe COPD (13/50 [26%]) compared with control subjects (3/50 [6%]) ($P = .01$).

Clinical Impact of Patent Foramen Ovale in Chronic Obstructive Pulmonary Disease

COPD can, in theory, worsen right-to-left shunting through a PFO. As COPD worsens in severity, patients experience increased respiratory loads, which can cause large swings in intrathoracic pressure, thereby increasing positive end-expiratory pressure.[68,69] Furthermore, acute exacerbations of COPD can cause PAP to rise.[69,70] These mechanisms, together, can potentially result in an increase in right atrial pressures and consequent right-to-left shunting. Accordingly, investigators sought out whether the presence of a PFO worsens hypoxemia as well as PAP and functional parameters, such as quality of life and exercise capacity, in COPD patients.

Soliman and colleagues[64], Shaikh and colleagues[68], and Kilic and colleagues[66] noted no significant difference in hypoxemia between COPD patients with and without PFO, while Hacievliyagil

and colleagues[65] and Martolini and colleagues[67] noted significantly worse hypoxemia in COPD patients with PFO than those without. This discrepancy may be explained by the existence of a concomitant intrapulmonary shunt at varying degrees of severity. For instance, Shaikh and colleagues[68] noted a significantly lower Pa_{O_2} in COPD patients that had an intrapulmonary shunt in addition to a PFO.

Both Soliman and colleagues[64] and Kilic and colleagues[66] observed that COPD patients with PFO had significantly higher pulmonary artery systolic pressures (PASPs). Soliman and colleagues[64] reported a higher degree of transient systemic arterial desaturation in COPD patients with PFO than those without ($-3.1 \pm 1.4\%$ vs $-1.5 \pm 0.5\%$, $P<.05$). However, they also noted that COPD patients displayed a similar trend with the Valsalva maneuver compared to normal subjects ($-2.6 \pm 1.4\%$ vs $-1.1 \pm 0.9\%$, $P<.005$), raising the issue of whether the presence of a PFO was the sole cause of the hypoxemia. Furthermore, the observed hypoxemia due to interatrial shunting through a PFO appeared to correlate with the degree of pulmonary hypertension (r = 0.6, $P<.05$). On the contrary, Hacievliyagil and colleagues[65] noted no significant difference in PASP among COPD patients with PFO and without PFO.

Assessing quality of life in COPD patients with PFO versus without PFO using the modified Medical Research Council dyspnea and St. George's Respiratory Questionnaire (SGRQ) scores yielded no significant differences in patient-reported symptom burden.[65–68] However, Shaikh and colleagues[68] reported lower SGRQ scores, which corresponds with better perceived overall well-being, in patients with severe COPD and PFO than those without.

Current research suggests that the presence of PFO does not negatively impact exercise performance. COPD patients with and without PFO subjected to cardiopulmonary exercise testing via cycle ergometry showed no significant differences in peak minute ventilation, maximal oxygen consumption adjusted for body weight, ratio of minute ventilation per unit of carbon dioxide at peak exercise, peak heart rate, and peak workload despite displaying signs of abdominal muscle recruitment to combat respiratory fatigue.[67,68] However, some subjects with PFO did demonstrate an increase in shunt size or worse hypoxemia with exercise, presumably due to increased right-to-left shunting, but these changes did not drastically worsen overall exercise performance.[67,68] Additionally, 6-minute walk distances (6MWD) generally did not differ between PFO and non-PFO groups, but Shaikh and colleagues[68] noted significantly

Table 2
Comparison of hypoxemia, pulmonary artery systolic pressures, and functional parameters in chronic obstructive pulmonary disease patients with and without patent foramen ovale

Reference	Number of Patients		Hypoxemia			Pulmonary Artery Systolic Pressure			Functional Parameters		
	With PFO	Without PFO	With PFO	Without PFO	P-Value	With PFO	Without PFO	P-Value	With PFO	Without PFO	P-Value
Soliman et al,[3] 1999	14	6	SaO2: 94 ± 2.1%	SaO2: 94 ± 2.3%	NS	38.3 ± 7.3 mm Hg	21.0 ± 2.4 mm Hg	P<.005			
Hacievliyagil et al,[4] 2006	23	29	Pao$_2$: 55.3 ± 10.9 mm Hg SaO2: 87.7 ± 6.9%	Pao$_2$: 63.3 ± 11.5 mm Hg SaO2: 91.7 ± 5.6%	P = .016 P = .041	57.6 ± 22.7 mm Hg	46.6 ± 13.8 mm Hg	NS	mMRC: 3.04 ± 0.88 6MWD: 315 ± 147 m	mMRC: 2.86 ± 0.99 6MWD: 386 ± 156 m	NS NS
Kilic et al,[5] 2010	4	17	Pao$_2$: 46.5 ± 13.7 mm Hg SaO2: 79.3 ± 12.8%	Pao$_2$: 57.4 ± 6.8 mm Hg SaO2: 90 ± 3.2%	NS NS	42.5 ± 6.5 mm Hg	33.8 ± 5.4 mm Hg	P = .031			
Martolini et al,[6] 2014	12	10	Pao$_2$: 10.1 ± 1.1 kPa SaO2: 96 ± 0.8%	Pao$_2$: 11.6 ± 0.8 kPa SaO2: 97 ± 0.64%	P = .0051 P = .0008				mMRC: 1.92 ± 0.9 SGRQ: 34 ± 12 6MWD: 485 ± 121 m	mMRC: 1.7 ± 0.67 SGRQ: 39 ± 23 6MWD: 492 ± 46 m	NS NS NS
Shaikh et al,[7] 2014	23	27	Pao$_2$: 8.6 kPa	Pao$_2$: 8.5 kPa	NS				6MWD: 312 m	6MWD: 243 m	P = .01

Data listed as mean values with standard deviation as available.
Abbreviations: 6MWD, 6-minute walk distance; mMRC, modified Medical Research Council dyspnea score; NS, not significant; Pao$_2$, partial pressure of oxygen in arterial blood; PFO, patent foramen ovale; SaO2, systemic arterial oxygen saturation; SGRQ, St. George's Respiratory Questionnaire score.

better 6MWD in severe COPD patients with PFO than those without (312 m vs 243 m, $P = .01$).[65,67]

Table 2 summarizes the findings on hypoxemia, PAPs, and functional parameters in COPD patients with and without PFO.

Outcomes of Percutaneous Patent Foramen Ovale Closure in Chronic Obstructive Pulmonary Disease

Some of the aforementioned observational studies suggest that PFOs do not impart a significant pathologic role in COPD, and therefore, screening for and closure of PFOs may not be clinically required. However, there have been case series that demonstrated improvement in supplemental oxygen requirements and dyspnea in patients with chronic lung disease of any type following percutaneous PFO closure.[71–73] In addition, case reports of patients with COPD and PFO undergoing PFO closure also share similar successful clinical endpoints.

Layoun and colleagues[74] described a 61-year-old male with moderate COPD and tobacco use disorder who demonstrated oxygen saturations of 84% to 88% at rest and 70% to 77% with exercise on room air and a 6MWD of 363 m. Since moderate COPD could not cause this degree of hypoxemia and functional impairment, a workup for alternative causes of hypoxemia was initiated. Accordingly, the patient underwent transesophageal echocardiogram, which showed a moderate-sized PFO, and this finding was confirmed on intracardiac echocardiography. Following percutaneous PFO closure, resting oxygen saturation improved to 91% to 92%, exercise oxygen saturation improved to 84%, and 6MWD improved to 422 m.

In a second case discussed by Layoun and colleagues[74], a 59-year-old morbidly obese male with asthma with COPD overlap of moderate severity and OSA treated with nightly CPAP machine presented with gradually worsening symptomatic hypoxemia. Oxygen saturation at rest on room air was 94%, and it declined to 87% with mild exertion. Given that the severity of hypoxemia was out of proportion to the severity of the underlying lung diseases, a TEE was performed, and it revealed a PFO. The patient underwent percutaneous PFO closure, and this alleviated his symptoms and improved oxygen saturation on room air to 94% with exercise.

Frizzelli and colleagues[75] described an 80-year-old male with unclassified COPD and former tobacco use who presented with chronic cough and dyspnea. Oxygen saturation on room air decreased from 90% to 78% and Pao$_2$ worsened from 54.8 mm Hg to 37 mm Hg when changing from the supine to upright position. Consequently, the patient was diagnosed with POS. Chest radiograph revealed spinal deviation. Transthoracic echocardiogram revealed thoracic aortic ectasia, a large Eustachian valve, and an estimated PASP of 40 mm Hg. Contrast TEE revealed an 11-mm PFO, and percutaneous PFO closure resulted in abolition of hypoxemia and ability to perform moderate exercise.

Summary and Future Directions

Although PFO may worsen the hypoxemia and elevated PAPs associated with COPD, it does not appear to significantly impair the quality of life or exercise performance.

Regardless, a handful of case series exist demonstrating an improvement in exertional hypoxemia and associated symptoms following percutaneous PFO closure in COPD patients. However, it should be noted that many of these reports lacked long-term follow-up, an adequate sample size, and a standardized methodology for detecting and quantifying PFOs. Furthermore, COPD is a heterogeneous disease, and as a result, it is difficult to distinguish the clinical and physiologic impact of this respiratory disease from that of the PFO. To help address this limitation, it would have been useful to measure the degree of intrapulmonary shunting. Lastly, the studies discussed did not indicate whether COPD treatment was optimized or quantify the severity of the emphysema. These missing variables may increase the role that COPD plays in causing hypoxemia and a decrease in functional parameters, thereby leading to the argument that PFO plays a small to irrelevant role.

In summary, further studies are needed to better address the aforementioned challenges and shortcomings and to clarify the role of percutaneous PFO closure in COPD patients with hypoxemia out of proportion to the underlying lung disease and PFO.

CLINICS CARE POINTS

- When evaluating for hypoxemia, consider PFO.
- If considering PFO as the cause of the underlying hypoxemia, perform a screening TCD instead of a transthoracic or transesophageal echocardiogram.
- Once a PFO is diagnosed, consult with local experts within and outside of cardiology to assess whether closing the interatrial shunt is in the best interest of the patient.

DISCLOSURES

None.

SUPPLEMENTARY DATA

Supplementary data to this article can be found online at https://doi.org/10.1016/j.ccl.2024.01.008.

REFERENCES

1. Burchell HB. Reflex orthostatic dyspnea associated with pulmonary hypotension. Am J Physiol 1949; 159:563–4.

2. Kamel M, Malik A, Sarkar K, et al. Orthodeoxia platypnea syndrome in the setting of cholangiocarcinoma: a case report. Am J Cardiol 2023;204: 64–9.

3. Sitbon S, Ou P, Nguyen C, et al. Four-dimensional flow magnetic resonance imaging features of a platypnea-orthodeoxia syndrome caused by a patent foramen ovale. Circ Cardiovasc Imaging 2023; 16(7):601–3.

4. Soares PR, Melo N, Ferrao D, et al. Platypnea-orthodeoxia syndrome: a rare cause of positional respiratory failure. Cureus 2022;14(12):e32538.

5. Alotaibi FF, Alotaibi RM, Almalki ME, et al. Patent foramen ovale-induced platypnea-orthodeoxia syndrome: a case report and literature review. Cureus 2022;14(12):e32203.

6. Mojadidi MK, Gevorgyan R, Noureddin N, et al. The effect of patent foramen ovale closure in patients with platypnea-orthodeoxia syndrome. Cathet Cardiovasc Interv 2015;86(4):701–7.

7. Shah AH, Osten M, Leventhal A, et al. Percutaneous intervention to treat platypnea-orthodeoxia syndrome: the Toronto experience. JACC Cardiovasc Interv 2016;9(18):1928–38.

8. Blanche C, Noble S, Roffi M, et al. Platypnea-orthodeoxia syndrome in the elderly treated by percutaneous patent foramen ovale closure: a case series and literature review. Eur J Intern Med 2013;24(8): 813–7.

9. Pristipino C, Germonpré P, Toni D, et al. European position paper on the management of patients with patent foramen ovale. Part II - decompression sickness, migraine, arterial deoxygenation syndromes and select high-risk clinical conditions. Eur Heart J 2021;42(16):1545–53.

10. Kavinsky CJ, Szerlip M, Goldsweig AM, et al. SCAI guidelines for the management of patent foramen ovale. J Soc Cardiovascul Angiograph Intervent 2022;1(4):100039.

11. Küçükseymen S, Ciardetti N, Stolcova M, et al. Platypnea-orthodeoxia syndrome following transcatheter aortic valve replacement. Anatol J Cardiol 2023;27(9):549–51.

12. Chopard R, Meneveau N. Right-to-left atrial shunting associated with aortic root aneurysm: a case report of a rare cause of platypnea-orthodeoxia syndrome. Heart Lung Circ 2013;22(1):71–5.

13. Eicher JC, Bonniaud P, Baudouin N, et al. Hypoxaemia associated with an enlarged aortic root: a new syndrome? Heart 2005;91(8):1030–5.

14. Han HJ, Lee J, Kim Y. An unusual cause of positional hypoxemia: platypnea-orthodeoxia syndrome caused by patent foramen ovale and ascending aortic dilatation. Eur Heart J Cardiovasc Imaging 2023. https://doi.org/10.1093/ehjci/jead267. jead267.

15. Laybourn KA, Martin ET, Cooper RA, et al. Platypnea and orthodeoxia: shunting associated with an aortic aneurysm. J Thorac Cardiovasc Surg 1997;113(5): 955–6.

16. Medina A, de Lezo JS, Caballero E, et al. Platypnea-orthodeoxia due to aortic elongation. Circulation 2001;104(6):741.

17. Molina-Lopez VH, Diaz-Rodriguez PE, Aviles-Rivera E, et al. Cardiac platypnea-orthodeoxia syndrome: a rare case of flow-directed, right-to-left shunt via a patent foramen ovale exacerbated by aortic root enlargement. Cureus 2023;15(8):e43721.

18. Savage EB, Benckart DH, Donahue BC, et al. Intermittent hypoxia due to right atrial compression by an ascending aortic aneurysm. Ann Thorac Surg 1996; 62(2):582–3.

19. Hamid K, Perinkulam Sathyanarayanan S, Hoerschgen K, et al. Right atrial thrombus presenting as platypnea-orthodeoxia secondary to reverse lutembacher syndrome: a case report. Cureus 2022;14(7):e26754.

20. Courtis J, Marani L, Amuchastegui LM, et al. Cardiac lipoma: a rare cause of right-to-left interatrial shunt with normal pulmonary artery pressure. J Am Soc Echocardiogr 2004;17(12):1311–4.

21. Wright RS, Simari RD, Orszulak TA, et al. Eosinophilic endomyocardial disease presenting as cyanosis, platypnea, and orthodeoxia. Ann Intern Med 1992;117(6):482–3.

22. Bokhari SSI, Willens HJ, Lowery MH, et al. Orthodeoxia platypnea syndrome in a patient with lipomatous hypertrophy of the interatrial septum due to long-term steroid use. Chest 2011;139(2):443–5.

23. Maniscalco M, Dialetto G, Tufano G, et al. Orthodeoxia without platypnea from interatrial defect associated with persistent left superior vena cava in the absence of pulmonary hypertension. Respiration 2003;70(2):207–10.

24. Rao P, Undavalli C, Ghoweba M, et al. Platypnea orthodeoxia syndrome secondary to a persistent eustachian valve. Cureus 2023;15(8):e42900.

25. Hsu PF, Leu HB, Lu TM, et al. Platypnea-orthodeoxia syndrome occurring after a blunt chest trauma with acute tricuspid regurgitation. Am J Med 2004; 117(11):890–1.

26. Somers C, Slabbynck H, Paelinck BP. Echocardio-graphic diagnosis of platypnoea-orthodeoxia syndrome after blunt chest trauma. Acta Cardiol 2000; 55(3):199–201.

27. Sakagianni K, Evrenoglou D, Mytas D, et al. Platypnea-orthodeoxia syndrome related to right hemidiaphragmatic elevation and a "stretched" patent foramen ovale. Case Reports 2012;2012. bcr-2012-007735-bcr-2012-007735.

28. Patakas D, Pitsiou G, Philippou D, et al. Reversible platypnoea and orthodeoxia after surgical removal of an hydatid cyst from the liver. Eur Respir J 1999;14(3):725.

29. Teupe CHJ, Groenefeld GC. Platypnea-orthodeoxia due to osteoporosis and severe kyphosis: a rare cause for dyspnea and hypoxemia. Heart Int 2011; 6(2). hi.2011.e13.

30. Vallurupalli S, Lodha A, Kupfer Y, et al. Platypnea-Orthodeoxia syndrome after repair of a paraesophageal hernia. BMJ Case Rep 2013;2013. bcr2012007444.

31. Mashman WE, Silverman ME. Platypnea related to constrictive pericarditis. Chest 1994;105(2):636–7.

32. Vora SG, Nierman DM. Platypnea related to constrictive pericarditis. Chest 1995;107(3):887.

33. Adolph EA, Lacy WO, Hermoni YI, et al. Reversible orthodeoxia and platypnea due to right-to-left intracardiac shunting related to pericardial effusion. Ann Intern Med 1992;116(2):138–9.

34. Roos CM, Romijn KH, Braat MC, et al. Posture-dependent dyspnea and cyanosis after pneumonectomy. Eur J Respir Dis 1981;62(6):377–82.

35. Salvetti M, Zotti D, Bazza A, et al. Platypnea and orthodeoxia in a patient with pulmonary embolism. Am J Emerg Med 2013;31(4):760.e1–2.

36. Khan F, Parekh A. Reversible platypnea and orthodeoxia following recovery from adult respiratory distress syndrome. Chest 1979;75(4):526–8.

37. Furuta Y, Sugahara M, Nakamura T, et al. Platypnea-orthodeoxia: an effective diagnostic tool for hepatopulmonary syndrome with chronic obstructive pulmonary disease. Cureus 2023;15(3):e35904.

38. Bourke SJ, Munro NC, White JE, et al. Platypnoea-orthodeoxia in cryptogenic fibrosing alveolitis. Respir Med 1995;89(5):387–9.

39. Takhar R, Biswas R, Arora A, et al. Platypnoea-orthodeoxia syndrome: novel cause for a known condition. Case Reports 2014;2014. bcr2013201284-bcr2013201284.

40. Bakris NC, Siddiqi AJ, Fraser CD, et al. Right-to-left interatrial shunt after pneumonectomy. Ann Thorac Surg 1997;63(1):198–201.

41. Begin R. Platypnea after pneumonectomy. N Engl J Med 1975;293(7):342–3.

42. Bhattacharya K, Birla R, Northridge D, et al. Platypnea-orthodeoxia syndrome: a rare complication after right pneumonectomy. Ann Thorac Surg 2009;88(6): 2018–9.

43. Papiris SA, Maniati MA, Manoussakis MN, et al. Orthodeoxia in amiodarone-induced acute reversible pulmonary damage. Chest 1994;105(3):965–6.

44. Gacad G. Orthostatic hypoxemia in a patient with bronchogenic carcinoma. Arch Intern Med 1974; 134(6):1113.

45. Ferry TG, Naum CC. Orthodeoxia-platypnea due to diabetic autonomic neuropathy. Diabetes Care 1999;22(5):857–9.

46. Gourgiotis S, Aloizos S, Gakis C, et al. Platypnea-orthodeoxia due to fat embolism. Int J Surg Case Reports 2011;2(6):147–9.

47. DesJardin JA, Martin RJ. Platypnea in the intensive care unit. A newly described cause. Chest 1993; 104(4):1308–9.

48. Bouros D, Agouridakis P, Tsatsakis A, et al. Orthodeoxia and platypnoea after acute organophosphorus poisoning reversed by CPAP: a newly described cause and review of the literature. Respir Med 1995;89(9):625–8.

49. Hussain SF, Mekan SF. Platypnea-orthodeoxia: report of two cases and review of the literature. South Med J 2004;97(7):657–62.

50. Awan AN, Ashraf R, Meyerson MB, et al. Radiation-induced bronchial stenosis: a new cause of platypnea-orthodeoxia. South Med J 1999;92(7):720–4.

51. Odell JA, Keller CA, Erasmus DB, et al. Traumatic bronchial rupture and platypnea-orthodeoxia. Ann Thorac Surg 2012;93(2):662–4.

52. Young T, Palta M, Dempsey J, et al. Burden of sleep apnea: rationale, design, and major findings of the Wisconsin Sleep Cohort study. Wis Med J 2009; 108(5):246–9.

53. Shanoudy H, Soliman A, Raggi P, et al. Prevalence of patent foramen ovale and its contribution to hypoxemia in patients with obstructive sleep apnea. Chest 1998;113(1):91–6.

54. Beelke M, Angeli S, Del Sette M, et al. Prevalence of patent foramen ovale in subjects with obstructive sleep apnea: a transcranial Doppler ultrasound study. Sleep Med 2003;4(3):219–23.

55. Mojadidi MK, Bokhoor PI, Gevorgyan R, et al. Sleep apnea in patients with and without a right-to-left shunt. J Clin Sleep Med 2015;11(11):1299–304.

56. Johansson MC, Eriksson P, Peker Y, et al. The influence of patent foramen ovale on oxygen desaturation in obstructive sleep apnoea. Eur Respir J 2006;29(1):149–55.

57. Loke YK, Brown JWL, Kwok CS, et al. Association of obstructive sleep apnea with risk of serious cardiovascular events: a systematic review and meta-analysis. Circ Cardiovasc Qual Outcomes 2012;5(5): 720–8.

58. Xie C, Zhu R, Tian Y, et al. Association of obstructive sleep apnoea with the risk of vascular outcomes and all-cause mortality: a meta-analysis. BMJ Open 2017;7(12):e013983.

59. Silver B, Greenbaum A, McCarthy S. Improvement in sleep apnea associated with closure of a patent foramen ovale. J Clin Sleep Med 2007;3(3):295–6.

60. Rimoldi SF, Ott S, Rexhaj E, et al. Patent foramen ovale closure in obstructive sleep apnea improves blood pressure and cardiovascular function. Hypertension 2015;66(5):1050–7.

61. Culpepper DJ, Hong D, Ryden A, et al. A 38-year-old man with well treated OSA on CPAP with persistent nocturnal hypoxemia. Chest 2020;157(1):e1–3.

62. Agustí A, Celli BR, Criner GJ, et al. Global initiative for chronic obstructive lung disease 2023 report: GOLD executive summary. Am J Respir Crit Care Med 2023;207(7):819–37.

63. Stanojevic S, Kaminsky DA, Miller MR, et al. ERS/ATS technical standard on interpretive strategies for routine lung function tests. Eur Respir J 2022; 60(1):2101499.

64. Soliman A, Shanoudy H, Liu J, et al. Increased prevalence of patent foramen ovale in patients with severe chronic obstructive pulmonary disease. J Am Soc Echocardiogr 1999;12(2):99–105.

65. Hacievliyagil SS, Gunen H, Kosar FM, et al. Prevalence and clinical significance of a patent foramen ovale in patients with chronic obstructive pulmonary disease. Respir Med 2006;100(5):903–10.

66. Kilic H, Balci MM, Aksoy MN, et al. Patent foramen ovale among patients with mild chronic obstructive pulmonary disease and unexplained hypoxia. Echocardiography 2010;27(6):687–90.

67. Martolini D, Tanner R, Davey C, et al. Significance of patent foramen ovale in patients with GOLD stage II chronic obstructive pulmonary disease (COPD). Chronic Obstr Pulm Dis 2014;1(2):185–92.

68. Shaikh ZF, Kelly JL, Shrikrishna D, et al. Patent foramen ovale is not associated with hypoxemia in severe chronic obstructive pulmonary disease and does not impair exercise performance. Am J Respir Crit Care Med 2014;189(5):540–7.

69. Boerrigter BG, Boonstra A, Westerhof N, et al. Cardiac shunt in COPD as a cause of severe hypoxaemia: probably not so uncommon after all. Eur Respir J 2011;37(4):960–2.

70. Chaouat A, Naeije R, Weitzenblum E. Pulmonary hypertension in COPD. Eur Respir J 2008;32(5):1371–85.

71. Fenster BE, Carroll JD. Patent foramen ovale in COPD and hypoxia: innocent bystander or novel therapeutic target? Chronic Obstr Pulm Dis 2014; 1(2):151–4.

72. Fenster BE, Nguyen BH, Buckner JK, et al. Effectiveness of percutaneous closure of patent foramen ovale for hypoxemia. Am J Cardiol 2013;112(8): 1258–62.

73. Ilkhanoff L, Naidu SS, Rohatgi S, et al. Transcatheter device closure of interatrial septal defects in patients with hypoxia. J Intervent Cardiol 2005;18(4):227–32.

74. Layoun ME, Aboulhosn JA, Tobis JM. Potential role of patent foramen ovale in exacerbating hypoxemia in chronic pulmonary disease. Tex Heart Inst J 2017; 44(3):189–97.

75. Frizzelli R, Lettieri C, Caiola S, et al. Unexplained hypoxemia in COPD with cardiac shunt. Respir Med Case Rep 2022;37:101661.

Patent Foramen Ovale and Acute Mountain Sickness

Brian West, MD[a], Jonathan M. Tobis, MD[b],*

KEYWORDS

- Patent foramen ovale • Right-to-left shunt • Acute mountain sickness
- High-altitude pulmonary edema

KEY POINTS

- Acute mountain sickness is thought to result from tissue hypoxia and can cause life-threatening illness in those who travel to high altitudes.
- Patent foramen ovale (PFO) is associated with right-to-left shunt and can worsen tissue hypoxia.
- PFO is an independent risk factor for developing acute mountain sickness and high-altitude pulmonary edema.

The history of acute mountain sickness (AMS) dates back at least 2000 years with a written report from the Chinese Han dynasty warning the Emperor Chung Ti against traveling over the Kilik Pass in the Karakorum Mountains at 4827 m (15,837 ft), which was a trade route between China and Afghanistan, because of the risk of getting sick.[1] The report states, "Next, one comes to Big Headache and Little Headache Mountains they make a man so hot that his face turns pale, his head aches, and he begins to vomit. Even the donkeys and swine react this way."

Mountain sickness is currently described by the Lake Louise Criteria, but still relies heavily on the subjective presence of headache, and gastrointestinal distress of anorexia, nausea, and vomiting. Hackett and coworkers[2] in the 1970s described 278 hikers who climbed from the airport at Lukla at 2800m to the Everest basecamp at 5356m without acclimating during their climb. Over 50% of climbers who ascended rapidly developed symptoms of AMS. In 1993, Honigman[3] described that 25% of tourists in Colorado who ascended to relatively lower altitudes of 6300 ft to 9700 ft developed mountain sickness. The most common complaints were headache (62%), insomnia (31%), fatigue (26%), shortness of breath (21%), dizziness (21%), loss of appetite (11%), and vomiting (3%).

Additionally in 1993, a consensus committee of respiratory physiologists met at Lake Louise, Canada and developed criteria for making the diagnosis of AMS.[4] **Fig. 1** presents the original criteria; a score of 3 or more was indicative of a diagnosis of AMS. The Lake Louise Criteria were revised in 2018 and sleep disturbance was removed because (1) subsequent data showed that sleep disturbance correlated poorly with the other variables and (2) many studies of AMS have included only daytime exposures. Instead of sleep disturbance, a functional grading was added to assess the severity of the symptoms.[5] **Fig. 2** provides the updated criteria. In this scale, AMS was considered to be mild with a score of 3 to 5, moderate with a score of 6 to 9, and severe with a score of 10 to 12.

A review article in the *New England Journal of Medicine* in 2013 by Bärtsch[6] described the continuum of altitude sickness from the symptoms of AMS to the development of high-altitude pulmonary edema (HAPE) and eventually high-altitude cerebral edema. Several authors describe the independent factors that may predispose to AMS, which include a prior history of AMS, days at altitude during the prior 2 months, and the rate of ascent.[7,8]

The proposed mechanism of AMS is that the decrease in the partial pressure of oxygen with

a Sharp Rees-Stealy Medical Group; b Ronald Reagan UCLA Medical Center
* Corresponding author.
E-mail address: jtobis@mednet.ucla.edu

Cardiol Clin 42 (2024) 521–524
https://doi.org/10.1016/j.ccl.2024.01.009

1. Headache.
   0   No headache
   1   Mild headache
   2   Moderate headache
   3   Severe headache, incapacitating

2. Gastrointestinal symptoms.
   0   No gastrointestinal symptoms
   1   Poor appetite or nausea
   2   Moderate nausea or vomiting
   3   Severe nausea & vomiting, incapacitating

3. Fatigue and/or weakness.
   0   Not tired or weak
   1   Mild fatigue/weakness
   2   Moderate fatigue/weakness
   3   Severe fatigue/weakness, incapacitating

4. Dizziness/lightheadedness.
   0   Not dizzy
   1   Mild dizziness
   2   Moderate dizziness
   3   Severe dizziness, incapacitating

5. Difficulty sleeping.
   0   Slept as well as usual
   1   Did not sleep as well as usual
   2   Woke many times, poor night's sleep
   3   Could not sleep at all

Fig. 1. The original Lake Louise Criteria for acute mountain sickness.

increasing altitude produces progressive hypoxemia with subsequent tissue depletion of essential oxygen. In the lungs and brain, this causes dysfunction of the vascular endothelium, with release of fluid into the interstitial spaces resulting in pulmonary and cerebral edema.

The potential connection with PFO and altitude-related illness is that the right-to-left shunt associated with a PFO, especially during exertion and

Headache
0—None at all
1—A mild headache
2—Moderate headache
3—Severe headache, incapacitating
Gastrointestinal symptoms
0—Good appetite
1—Poor appetite or nausea
2—Moderate nausea or vomiting
3—Severe nausea and vomiting, incapacitating
Fatigue and/or weakness
0—Not tired or weak
1—Mild fatigue/weakness
2—Moderate fatigue/weakness
3—Severe fatigue/weakness, incapacitating
Dizziness/light-headedness
0—No dizziness/light-headedness
1—Mild dizziness/light-headedness
2—Moderate dizziness/light-headedness
3—Severe dizziness/light-headedness, incapacitating
AMS Clinical Functional Score
Overall, if you had AMS symptoms, how did they affect your activities?
0—Not at all
1—Symptoms present, but did not force any change in activity or itinerary
2—My symptoms forced me to stop the ascent or to go down on my own power
3—Had to be evacuated to a lower altitude

Fig. 2. The 2018 modified Lake Louise acute mountain sickness scale.

straining, could increase the hypoxemia, which would exacerbate the hypoxemia produced by the lower partial pressure of oxygen at higher altitudes.

To test the hypothesis that a patent foramen ovale (PFO) increases the likelihood of developing HAPE, Alleman and colleagues[9] studied 35 experienced mountain climbers; 16 had a history of developing HAPE and 19 climbers who had no history of HAPE. Transthoracic echocardiography with agitated saline was used to determine the presence of a right-to-left shunt. The investigators found that climbers with a history of HAPE had a markedly increased frequency of PFO, 69%, compared with 16% in the climbers without a history of HAPE ($P < .001$). The arterial saturation measured at 4560 m was 73% in the HAPE-susceptible climbers and 83% in the climbers who did not have an episode of HAPE. These observations are consistent with the hypothesis that a PFO predisposes to developing severe altitude illness.

The authors were suspicious that the same physiology might be present in the more common type of AMS. To test this hypothesis, the authors assessed the frequency of PFO in hikers in California's Sierra Nevada range who climbed over Mount Whitney (14,500 ft) after acclimating along the John Muir Trail (JMT) and hikers who did not acclimate but rapidly ascended Mount Whitney from the eastern escarpment at Whitney portal (8000 ft) (**Fig. 3**).

Subjects who had hiked to altitudes above 10,000 ft (»3000 m) were recruited to this study.

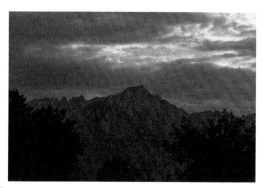

Fig. 3. Mount Whitney, California at 14,500 ft in the middle. Trail camp at 12,000 ft is at the base of Mt. Whitney above the level of the tree line.

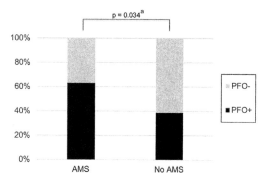

Fig. 4. Prevalence of PFO in the subjects with acute mountain sickness (AMS) and those subjects without AMS. [a]Comparison via Pearson $\chi 2$, significant at level $P < .05$.

The initial group had climbed all or part of the JMT in California. The JMT varies in altitude from 4000 ft in Yosemite Valley to 14,500 ft at the top of Mount Whitney. In 2015, the JMT Survey Group conducted a self-reported analysis of 1500 hikers.[10] These survey participants were asked to come to the University of California, Los Angeles to complete an AMS questionnaire and to undergo a transcranial Doppler (TCD) study.

To increase enrollment, a second method for recruiting subjects was devised. Permission was obtained from the Inyo National Forest Service to recruit hikers along the Mount Whitney Trail during the 2017 and 2018 summers. Recruiters were stationed both at Whitney Portal (8000 ft) and at Whitney Trail Camp (12,000 ft). Hikers were provided information about the study and were consented before participating. Volunteers were directed to the Southern Inyo Hospital in Lone Pine, California, in the Owens Valley below Mount Whitney. Upon arrival, they completed an AMS questionnaire. This included the original Lake Louise AMS Scoring System as well as questions regarding acclimatization and premedication, and whether climbers had to stop their ascent due to symptoms or if their symptoms were alleviated by descent.

During the initial recruitment phase as well as during the summers of 2017 and 2018, 137 hikers were recruited into the study.[11] Of these participants, 59 (43%) hikers were diagnosed with a PFO and 78 (57%) hikers were negative for a PFO. There were no significant baseline differences between these groups.

Based on adjudication before TCD testing, 24 (18%) hikers had symptoms consistent with AMS and 113 (82%) hikers did not. There was a higher prevalence of PFO in hikers with AMS, 15 of 24 (63%) compared with hikers without AMS, 44 of 113 (39%; **Fig. 4**). The presence of a PFO significantly increased the risk for developing AMS;

odds ratio 2.61, 95% confidence intervals 1.05 to 6.49; $P = .038$.

In the multivariate model, when adjusted for age, gender, AMS prophylaxis, and acclimatization, the relation between PFO and AMS became stronger: odds ratio 4.15, 95% confidence intervals 1.14 to 15.05; $P = .03$. None of the other variables in the model were significant predictors for AMS.

Lake Louise AMS Scores were significantly higher in hikers who were adjudicated as having AMS compared with those who were adjudicated as having no AMS, 7.43 ± 3.04 vs 2.89 ± 2.27, respectively; $P < .0001$. When the categories of "Difficulty Sleeping" and "Fatigue and/or Weakness" were removed, the scores remained significantly higher in the hikers who were adjudicated as having AMS compared with those who were adjudicated as having no AMS, 4.67 ± 1.32 vs 1.59 ± 1.49, respectively; $P < .0001$. TCD Spencer grade was significantly higher in those who developed AMS compared with those who did not develop AMS ($P = .011$; **Fig. 5**).

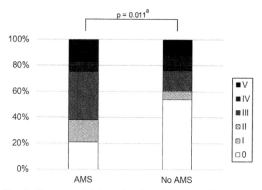

Fig. 5. Transcranial Doppler (TCD) degree of right-to-left shunting in subjects with acute mountain sickness (AMS) and those subjects without acute mountain sickness (No AMS). [a]Comparison via Fischer's exact test, significant at level $P < .05$.

If the development of AMS was solely related to right-to-left shunting, one would expect to see a significant difference in oxygen saturations between those who develop AMS and those who do not, particularly at high altitudes. The authors did not find this association but the oxygen saturation was obtained at rest at 12,000 ft, not during exercise. Additionally, there was a significant portion of participants with PFO in the authors' study who did not develop AMS. It is interesting to note there were a large number of hikers, both with and without AMS, who had a PFO in the authors' study. The prevalence in our population was 43%, which is higher than typical rates seen in other populations.[12,13] The reason for this is unclear.

The association between PFO and AMS does not prove causation; instead, our findings are hypothesis generating. Additional studies are needed to further elucidate the relation between PFO and AMS. Moreover, a prospective randomized trial of PFO closure versus standard therapy is warranted to determine whether PFO closure could alleviate the symptoms of AMS.

Clinicians should consider PFO a risk factor in patients who plan to hike to high altitudes.

CLINICS CARE POINTS

- When evaluating patients considering ascending to high altitudes, consider screening for PFO as a risk factor for AMS.
- In patients who develop AMS, consider screening for PFO.

DISCLOSURE

The authors have nothing to disclose.

REFERENCES

1. Gilbert DL. The first documented report of mountain sickness: the China or Headache Mountain story. Respir Physiol 1983;52(3):315–26.

2. Hackett PH, Rennie D, Levine HD. The incidence, importance, and prophylaxis of acute mountain sickness. Lancet 1976;2(7996):1149–55.

3. Honigman B, Theis MK, Koziol-McLain J, et al. Acute mountain sickness in a general tourist population at moderate altitudes. Ann Intern Med 1993;118(8):587–92.

4. Roach R, Bartsch P, Hacket P, et al. The Lake Louise Acute Mountain Sickness scoring System. Hypoxia and molecular medicine 1993;272–4.

5. Roach RC, Hackett PH, Oelz O, et al, Lake Louise AMS Score Consensus Committee. The 2018 Lake Louise Acute Mountain Sickness score. High Alt Med Biol 2018;19(1):4–6.

6. Bartsch P, Swenson E. Clinical practice: acute high-altitude illnesses. New England journal of medicine 2013;368(24):2294–302.

7. Schneider M, Bernasch D, Weymann J, et al. Acute mountain sickness: influence of susceptibility, preexposure, and ascent rate. Med Sci Sports Exerc 2002;34(12):1886–91.

8. Davis C, Hackett P. Advances in the prevention and treatment of high altitude illness. Emerg Med Clin North Am 2017;35(2):241–60.

9. Allemann Y, Hutter D, Lipp E, et al. Patent foramen ovale and high-altitude pulmonary edema. JAMA 2006;296(24):2954–8.

10. Rozier L, Aksamit I, Meyer K. An unofficial acclimatization guideline for JMT Hikers. 2015. https://unofficialacclimatizationguideline.blogspot.com/p/survey-results.html.

11. West BH, Fleming RG, Al Hemyari B, et al. Relation of patent foramen ovale to Acute Mountain Sickness. Am J Cardiol 2019;123(12):2022–5.

12. West BH, Noureddin N, Mamzhi Y, et al. Frequency of patent foramen ovale and migraine in patients with cryptogenic stroke. Stroke 2018;49(5):1123–8.

13. Khalid Mojadidi M, Scott C, et al. Accuracy of transcranial Doppler for the diagnosis of intracardiac right-to-left shunt: a bivariate meta-analysis of prospective studies. J Am Coll Cardiol Img 2014. https://doi.org/10.1016/j.jcmg.2013.12.011. Published online February 19.

Patent Foramen Ovale and Decompression Illness
The Present and Future

Sanjana Nagraj, MBBS[a], Leonidas Palaiodimos, MD, MS[b],*

KEYWORDS

- Decompression illness • Patent foramen ovale • Decompression sickness • Arterial gas embolism
- PFO • Diving • Hyperbaric oxygen

KEY POINTS

- Decompression sickness is the symptomatic involvement of one or more organ systems by bubbles released into tissues and blood vessels from a previously dissolved state.
- The presence of patent foramen ovale (PFO) increases the risk of developing decompression illness (DCI) and predisposes to more severe forms of DCI. However, not all divers with PFO develop DCI.
- Routine screening of all divers for PFO is not recommended. Indications for PFO screening are severe neurologic or cutaneous symptoms, or recurrent DCI, migraine with aura, DCI after a nonprovocative dive or DCI symptoms within 30 minutes of resurfacing.
- Recompression with hyperbaric oxygen forms the cornerstone treatment of DCI.
- In patients with established PFO-mediated DCI, ceasing diving or PFO closure and/or modifying diving practices to avoid provocative dives is recommended for the prevention of recurrent DCI.

INTRODUCTION

Decompression sickness (DCS) is the symptomatic involvement of one or more organ systems by bubbles released into tissues and blood vessels from a previously dissolved state, due to transition from a high-pressure environment to relatively lower pressures.[1] While traditionally linked with scuba diving, it can occur in any condition that involves rapid depressurization, such as during spacewalk in depressurized space suits and while flying in an unpressurized aircraft.[2] Arterial gas embolism is the entry of bubbles into the arterial circulation leading to end-organ ischemia, the etiology of which could be diving-related, pulmonary barotrauma, or iatrogenic. Due to similar clinical presentation and management protocols, DCS and arterial gas embolism are often consolidated under the common term decompression illness (DCI).

While the overall incidence of DCI is low, there is a wide fluctuation in its incidence, with recreational, instructor-led, military, and/or commercial diving carrying an incidence of 0.9 to 35.3 per 10,000 person-dives.[3] Among experienced scientific divers, the estimated incidence is much lower at 0.324 per 10,000 person-dives.[3] Despite a low incidence, the manifestations and clinical implications of DCI can be significant due to the organ systems involved, the extent or severity of involvement, and an increased propensity for severe phenotypes of DCI in the presence of structural

a Division of Cardiology, Montefiore Medical Center, Albert Einstein College of Medicine, 111 East 210th Street, Bronx, NY 10467, USA; b Department of Medicine, New York City Health + Hospitals/Jacobi, Albert Einstein College of Medicine, 1400 Pelham Parkway South, Bronx, NY 10461, USA
* Corresponding author. Department of Medicine, Jacobi Medical Center and Albert Einstein College of Medicine, 1400 Pelham Parkway South, Bronx, NY 10461.
E-mail address: leonidas.palaiodimos@gmail.com

Cardiol Clin 42 (2024) 525–536
https://doi.org/10.1016/j.ccl.2024.01.010

lesions.[4] The mechanism of DCI is due to super-saturation of tissues with dissolved gas at high external pressure. When the external pressure is relieved, such as by resurfacing from scuba diving, the soluble gas in the tissues enucleates and form bubbles that enter the arterial circulation, either through right-to-left shunts (intrapulmonary or intracardiac) or from pulmonary barotrauma. Venous gas emboli can also enter the arterial circulation by superseding the filtration capacity of the pulmonary capillary network.[5] Among lesions that can serve as right-to-left shunts, patent foramen ovale (PFO) takes precedence due to its wide prevalence in the general population. PFO is an intracardiac aperture due to persistence of the fetal structure foramen ovale into adulthood.[2] Allowing passage of blood from the right to the left atrium in the fetus, bypassing the pulmonary circulation, a persistent PFO is the most common congenital cardiac abnormality with a prevalence of 25% to 30% in the general population.[2] The risk of DCI and its debilitating forms such as neurologic DCI increases by 2.5 to 5 fold in the presence of PFO, which facilitates entry of bubbles into the arterial circulation.[6] A summary of the pathophysiology of DCI, subtypes with respective symptomatology, and commonly encountered DCI mimics precede a more extensive discussion of DCI in relation to PFO.

PATHOPHYSIOLOGY OF DECOMPRESSION ILLNESS

The risk of DCI increases with provocative dives, wherein the risk is directly related to the absolute depth of the dive, the amount of time spent at any given depth, and the rate of ascent toward lower ambient pressure. Similarly, in pilots, a rapid ascent into the lower pressure of high altitude is associated with the development of DCI.[5] Usually, nitrogen from divers' air tanks increases in partial pressure as the descent advances. For every 33 feet descent under water, the pressure increases by 11.6 pounds per inch (5.26 kg per 2.54 cm),[2] allowing more nitrogen to dissolve in tissues as the pressure increases.[5] With relatively rapid ascent that is out of proportion to the sheer volume of nitrogen dissolved in tissues, the dissolved gas is released as bubbles from tissues, either into the tissues or in the blood passing through them.[6] Typically, bubbles that enter the venous circulation are filtered from the bloodstream through pulmonary capillary diffusion and are exhaled. However, the overwhelming volume of bubbles released can exhaust the pulmonary filtration process and lead to florid DCI by entering the arterial circulation.[7] In patients with PFO, or another right-to-left shunt, nitrogen bubbles inconveniently bypass the suboptimal pulmonary filter and can cause systemic embolization, even in those who practice safe dives.[7]

SUBTYPES AND SYMPTOMATOLOGY
Type 1 Decompression Sickness

Musculoskeletal, cutaneous, and/or lymphatic system involvement form milder forms of Type 1 DCS.[5,8,9]

Musculoskeletal decompression illness
The musculoskeletal system is the most commonly involved organ system in those presenting with symptoms of DCI (50%–65% of patients) and as stated previously comprises one of its mildest forms.[5] Involvement is usually multifocal and affects shoulders, elbows, hips, and knees in a nonspecific manner. Secondary to the release of nitrogen bubbles into joints and muscles, patients describe a deep, dull ache that is not affected by movement and without localized tenderness.[5] Fatigue is a common symptom occurring to a degree out of proportion to the activity performed, particularly prominent when occurring in experienced divers.[8] A relevant consideration while evaluating patients with possible musculoskeletal DCI is trauma, the presentation of which is often unifocal and associated with discernible injury.[5] There appears to be no reported association between musculoskeletal DCI and PFO in current literature.

Cutaneous decompression illness
Cutaneous DCI also known as cutis marmorata presents as an erythematous, pruritic rash in an irregular distribution that progresses to skin mottling with a broken net-like pattern.[9] The pathognomonic rash gives the skin a bruised and marbled appearance. Although, the musculoskeletal system is considered to be most commonly involved in DCI, in a case series by Xu and colleagues with 5278 patients, cutaneous abnormalities were the most common symptoms, occurring in 65% of the cases.[10] Cutaneous DCI has been associated with right-to-left shunts, particularly PFO, because cutaneous manifestations are the result of arterial gas embolism.[11] In a small study by Hartig and colleagues, in 18 divers with DCI, all of the divers had a right-to-left shunt and 83% had a PFO. Cutaneous involvement, although not associated with serious sequalae, carries clinical significance, as it is one of the earliest signs of DCI.[12] Identification of cutaneous DCI can prompt urgent referral to a facility with hyperbaric oxygen for the evaluation and management of other potential severe manifestations.

Cutaneous DCI often resolves spontaneously within hours to days.

Lymphatic decompression illness

Lymphatic DCI is characterized by lymphadenopathy and lymphadenitis in a truncal distribution, especially in the upper chest and shoulders and occurs in 1% to 5% of the cases.[5] No studies reporting an association between lymphatic DCI and PFO were found.

Type 2 Decompression Sickness

Neurologic decompression illness

Across the wide spectrum of clinical presentation, neurologic involvement, especially when symptomatic, represents a more severe and debilitating form of DCI.[1,13] The presence of PFO or right-to-left shunt, especially when large, has been associated with the development of neurologic DCI, such as subclinical brain embolism with gradual decline in brain function and a variety of neurologic symptoms.[1,14,15] However, the absence of PFO or right-to-left shunt does not preclude their occurrence, and studies have shown that the act of diving by itself, in the absence of right-to-left shunt, has been associated with asymptomatic brain lesions.[14] In a recent meta-analysis by Peppas and colleagues of 1902 patients, of which 954 had neurologic DCI, the most common predisposing factors for the development of neurologic DCI were provocative diving techniques such as rapid ascent, missed stops for decompressions, violating prescribed table limits, repetitive diving, and concurrent lung disease.[1] In this study, 62.6% of divers with neurologic DCI had right-to-left shunt, compared to 27.3% of divers without neurologic DCI. Importantly, the investigators found divers with right-to-left shunt to carry a significantly higher odds (nearly 4-fold) of developing neurologic DCI compared to divers without right-to-left shunt (odds ratio [OR]: 3.83; 95% confidence interval [CI]: 2.79 to 5.27; $P < .001$).[1] This association was maintained on subgroup analysis, wherein right-to-left shunt was strongly associated with the development of both cerebral and spinal neurologic DCI.[1]

Inner ear decompression illness

Inner ear DCI is often considered a manifestation of neurologic DCI. Symptoms usually occur within 2 hours of surfacing and the presence of vertigo, ataxia, nausea, and vomiting suggest vestibular origin. Around 25% of patients experience cochlear symptoms such as hearing loss and tinnitus.[16] Based on 2346 cases of inner ear DCI reported to the Divers Alert Network, dizziness/vertigo occurred in 19.4%, coordination disturbance in 7.9%, and auditory symptoms in 2.1% of the patients.[17] The prevalence of PFO in patients with inner ear DCI is around 83%, and in the presence of a right-to-left shunt, there is an overwhelmingly increased risk of developing inner ear DCI (OR for developing inner ear DCI with right-to-left shunt: 12.13; 95% CI: 8.10–18.17 in a study of 244 divers with inner ear DCI).[1]

Cardiopulmonary decompression illness

A severe form of decompression illness, cardiopulmonary involvement typically occurs with provocative dives (violating table limits, rapid ascent, diving greater than 25 m, not stopping at designated times for decompression), and symptom onset is usually within 30 minutes of surfacing.[10] Cardiopulmonary decompression illness occurs in 1% to 5% of the cases and can present with arrhythmias, pulmonary edema, cough, chest pain, shock, and coagulopathy.[5] It is important to distinguish immersion pulmonary edema from cardiopulmonary DCI, wherein symptoms can occur before ascent with the former.

DECOMPRESSION ILLNESS AND PATENT FORAMEN OVALE
Factors Associated with Increased Risk of Decompression Illness in the Presence of Patent Foramen Ovale

The presence of PFO increases the risk of DCI by 2.5-fold to 5-fold, increases the risk of more severe forms of DCI and yet, not all divers with PFO develop DCI.[2] Equally important to note is that the occurrence of DCI, despite practicing safe diving techniques, can indicate an underlying PFO or another right-to-left shunt.[7,14] This corroborates with the fundamental mechanism by which PFO facilitates paradoxic embolism and stroke, wherein clots or bubbles can traverse from the venous to the arterial circulation.[18] In a prospective registry of 489 recreational divers, Honek and colleagues demonstrated that 97.2% of divers with unprovoked DCS had a PFO diagnosed by transcranial Doppler (TCD) compared to 35.5% of controls (recreational divers who did not develop DCS).[4] In the adjusted Cox proportional hazards model, high-grade PFO (PFO grade 3 as defined by the International Consensus Criteria) was a significant risk factor for unprovoked DCS.[4] Similarly, Lee and colleagues in their single-center prospective cohort study, found high-risk PFO, defined as either an atrial septal aneurysm or hypermobility, a PFO height of 2 mm or greater on TEE, and presence of shunting at rest, to be an independent risk factor for DCI (OR: 9.34; 95%CI: 1.95–44.88; $P = .005$).[19] In their study of 100 divers who did greater than 50 dives per year, 68% had a PFO, of which 54% had a high-risk PFO.[19] Subsequently, the incidence of DCI in the non-PFO group was 0 per 10,000 dives and 8.4 per 10,000 dives in the high-risk PFO group (P = .001).[19] Among those with PFO, factors associated with an increased risk of paradoxic embolism can be categorized as PFO-related factors (directly pertain to fundamental characteristics of the aperture) and factors that increase right heart pressures. Paradoxic embolism of bubbles in the presence of a PFO is illustrated in **Fig. 1**.

Patent foramen ovale-related factors

Large-sized/high-grade PFO with a wider diameter, larger shunt flow, high septal primum mobility, and spontaneous shunting increase the risk of DCI compared with subjects with smaller PFO.[6,20–22] High-grade PFO include those with greater than 100 microembolic signals in the middle cerebral artery on TCD using the Spencer's Logarithmic Scale (grade IV; 101–300 microembolic signals and grade V: >300 microembolic signals) or passage of greater than 20 microbubbles, cloud of microbubbles, or passage of contrast at rest on transthoracic echocardiogram (TTE) or transesophageal echocardiogram (TEE). In a study evaluating PFO size associated with DCI, Wilmhurst and colleagues found the median diameter of PFO in divers with a history of DCI to be 10 mm.[23] Factors associated with recurrence of DCI include not following diving protocols, and failure to reduce the time spent diving and depth of the dives apart from other listed factors.[24]

Conditions that increase right heart pressures

Cold-water immersion leads to peripheral vasoconstriction and subsequently increased venous return, which in turn raises right atrial pressure.[25] In the presence of a PFO, a relatively higher right atrial pressure facilitates shunting of the blood from right to left. Similarly, lifting heavy equipment at the end of the dive, performing a Valsalva maneuver to equalize middle ear pressure, bearing down, and excess entry of gas bubbles into the pulmonary filtration system can increase right-sided cardiac pressures and facilitate right-to-left shunting.[2,4,26]

ASYMPTOMATIC BRAIN LESIONS AND PATENT FORAMEN OVALE

Asymptomatic brain lesions are white-matter lesions seen as white-matter hyperintensities on both T2-weighted and fluid-attenuated inversion recovery MRI.[2] These lesions are believed to represent subclinical, cumulative ischemic damage to the brain and concerns regarding their

detrimental impact on long-term cognitive function exist.[27] Erdem and colleagues in their study of 113 military divers and 65 nondivers in apparent good health found a significantly higher number of brain lesions in military divers compared to nondivers (23% vs 11%; P = .04).[27] The investigators did not evaluate for underlying PFO in these groups. Balestra and colleagues reported a significant decline in higher cognitive function, visual-motor skills, and neuropsychiatric function in recreational divers with no association between asymptomatic brain lesions and PFO.[15] The investigators hypothesized the decline in cognitive function to nitrogen narcosis. Gempp and colleagues in their study of 32 asymptomatic military divers and 32 nondiving healthy subjects found a significantly higher number of cerebral hyperintensities in divers compared to the nondivers.[28] The investigators also found a positive correlation between asymptomatic brain lesions and the grade of right-to-left shunt.[28] However, the association of asymptomatic brain lesions with PFO is controversial in current literature due to a multitude of factors.[1,15] Taking multiple studies into consideration, around 40% of divers with asymptomatic brain lesions seen on MRI have been found to have PFO diagnosed by TCD.[15,28–31] Equally remarkable is the observation that nearly 40% of divers without asymptomatic brain lesions also have right-to-left shunt.[1,28,30,31] This is likely secondary to the widespread prevalence of right-to-left shunt, but this is 2 times the prevalence of PFO in the general population. The nearly equal distribution of PFO between those with and without asymptomatic brain lesions can explain the lack of significant association between PFO and asymptomatic brain lesions. Other factors contributing to the conflicting results include studies that could have been underpowered to detect a significant difference due to a small study population, an overall low incidence of diving pathology, and suboptimal study quality. For instance, in the study by Gerriets and colleagues in 42 sport divers, the authors could not confirm an association between asymptomatic brain lesions and the presence of right-to-left shunt.[29] However, in a recent well-conducted meta-analysis from 2023 evaluating healthy divers without a history of DCI, there was no significant association between presence of right-to-left shunt and asymptomatic brain lesions.[1] Controlled studies have also found that the act of diving by itself, in the absence of right-to-left shunt, increases the risk of detectable MRI signal abnormalities among military and recreational divers compared to nondiving healthy subjects.[14,27,28] Based on the evidence, it can be concluded that diving, irrespective of right-to-left shunt, is associated with

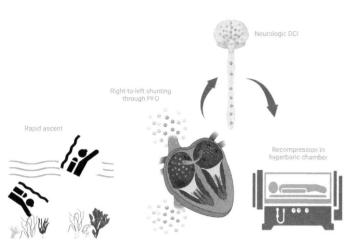

Fig. 1. Paradoxic embolism of bubbles through PFO resulting in right to left shunting.

Neurologic DCI

Right-to-left shunting through PFO

Rapid ascent

Recompression in hyperbaric chamber

an increased number of white-matter brain lesions, which may be implicated in long-term cognitive decline. However, causality cannot be established based on the available evidence.

PATIENT SELECTION FOR INVESTIGATING PATENT FORAMEN OVALE IN DIVERS

As 25% to 30% of the population has a PFO and the overall incidence of DCI is low, routine screening of all divers for PFO is not recommended across guidelines and consensus statements, including those released by the Undersea and Hyperbaric Medical Society and Health and Safety Executive from the United Kingdom.[32–34] Therefore, if a diver has not had DCI, routine evaluation for PFO should not be recommended, and rather, safe diving practices should be iterated.[34] In the case where a diver has had 1 episode of DCI, the following factors are suggestive of an underlying PFO and should be considered while deciding on PFO testing: severe DCI, neurologic or cutaneous DCI, migraine with aura, DCI after a nonprovocative dive, and DCI symptoms within 30 minutes of resurfacing.[34] If the diver engaged in a provocative dive that can explain the DCI, PFO testing is not indicated. If there is a history of recurrent DCI, PFO testing should be pursued.[34]

According to the National Oceanic and Atmospheric Administration (NOAA) diving medical standards and procedures manual published in 2010, an atrial septal defect, unless surgically corrected, is a disqualifying condition precluding safe diving.[32] However, PFO is not an absolute disqualifying condition and should be evaluated further for right-to-left shunting.[32] In divers with unprovoked decompression illness, testing for underlying PFO is indicated either with bubble contrast echocardiography or with TCD. In patients with

neurologic decompression illness and PFO, if the PFO is deemed to be a contributing factor after formal review, it is a disqualifying condition unless repaired as per the NOAA diving medical standards.[32] The Health and Safety Executive 2023 recommendation is in agreement with examination for PFO in patients with neurologic, cutaneous, or cardiopulmonary DCI, especially if there is a personal history of migraine with aura or a family history of PFO or atrial septal defect.[33] However, the presence of a PFO in these cases does not serve as an immediately disqualifying condition unless it is obvious that the diving profile was noncontributory to the DCI.[34] Further evaluation by a cardiologist with expertise in diving medicine is recommended in such cases, especially if the patient intends to continue diving. In patients with known PFO who are considering diving, it is important to evaluate for right-to-left shunting both at rest and with provocation for risk stratification. Provocative maneuvers such as Valsalva or sniffing should be used while performing echocardiography with bubble study. A PFO that exhibits right-to-left shunting with no or minimal provocation is a risk factor for severe DCI, particularly neurologic, inner ear, and cutaneous DCI.[1]

IMAGING TESTS FOR DETECTION OF PATENT FORAMEN OVALE

A PFO can be diagnosed in most instances using an echocardiogram, TTE or TEE or using TCD of the middle cerebral artery.[35] In the echocardiographic literature, TEE is considered the gold standard investigation for diagnosing PFO; however, there is a 10% false-negative rate with TEE, often because a Valsalva maneuver is significantly harder to perform while the TEE probe is in the patient's oropharynx and esophagus.[2] We prefer a gold standard of a right heart catheterization with the demonstration of passing a catheter across the atrial septum into the left atrium. Ideally, all echo bubble studies should be compared with that to determine sensitivity and specificity. Use of agitated saline to form bubbles, ideally pushed through the antecubital vein, both at rest (to detect spontaneous right-to-left shunting) and during provocative maneuvers such as Valsalva (inducible right-to-left shunting) is important to detect the PFO and grade the severity of the right-to-left shunt.[36] Visualization of agitated saline bubbles by TCD of the middle cerebral artery is also diagnostic of a right-to-left shunt. However, TCD cannot accurately detect the level of the right-to-left shunt (PFO vs atrial septal defect vs pulmonary arteriovenous shunt), although in the UCLA (University of California, Los Angeles) experience with 1500 TCD studies, the incidence of a pulmonary arteriovenous malformation was only 1%; 99% of the time the right-to-left shunt is due to a PFO.[37]

INTERVENTIONS FOR PATENT FORAMEN OVALE-MEDIATED DECOMPRESSION ILLNESS

In patients with established PFO-mediated decompression illness, ceasing diving or PFO repair and/or modifying diving practices to avoid provocative dives is recommended for the prevention of recurrent DCI.[2,34] Shared decision-making should be made in conjunction with a cardiologist with expertise in diving medicine in respect to continued diving and PFO closure. Although there have been studies conducted in small groups of divers who have undergone PFO closure, according to the 2010 National Institute of Clinical Excellence guidelines current evidence on the efficacy of percutaneous PFO closure for secondary prevention of paradoxic embolism in divers is inadequate and procedure efficacy is unknown in this population.[38] There is observational evidence that PFO closure is effective.

In a small case series of 28 divers with a history of neurologic DCI treated with percutaneous PFO closure, 23 returned to diving and had no recurrence of DCI.[38] In the DIVE-PFO prospective registry, Honek and colleagues compared the incidence of unprovoked DCI in 55 divers who underwent catheter-based PFO closure (indication for closure: grade 3 PFO and either a history of unprovoked DCI or diver preference) versus 98 divers with grade 3 PFO who were recommended conservative diving practices.[39] Over a mean (SD) follow-up of 7.1 (±3.8) years, none of the divers in the PFO closure group developed DCI while 11% of divers developed DCI in the conservative group

$(P = .012).$[39] The complication rate was minimal with 2 patients developing minor bleeding after PFO closure. Similarly, in another study, Honek and colleagues demonstrated the efficacy of catheter-based PFO closure in simulated diving conditions, wherein none of the divers who underwent PFO closure had arterial bubbles on TCD compared to 88% of divers with high-grade PFO.[40] Based on the findings of these 2 studies, the investigators concluded that PFO closure should be performed in divers with a high-grade PFO who have a history of unprovoked DCS or at the diver's preference (commercial divers for whom nonprovocative dives are nonnegotiable).[39] In a meta-analysis of 309 divers, of whom 141 underwent PFO closure, over a mean follow-up duration of 6.12 years (SD ± 0.70), the relative risk (RR) of DCI with PFO closure was significantly lower (RR: 0.29; 95% CI: 0.10–0.89) with a number needed to treat of 11, compared to divers who did not undergo PFO closure.[41] The incidence of complications was 7.63% in this study.[41] After PFO closure, echocardiogram or TCD with bubble study should be performed at 3 months to confirm satisfactory PFO closure and shunt elimination before resuming diving.[42] **Table 1** summarizes key studies on PFO closure in patients with DCI.

Conservative diving profile: In patients with PFO and unprovoked DCI, conservative diving practices can be used as an intermediary option between complete cessation of diving and PFO closure.[5,34] Diving to a depth less than 15 m, finishing the deepest part of the dive first, using Nitrox or another mixture with a relatively lower percentage of nitrogen to decrease the total nitrogen load, minimizing the use of Valsalva maneuver, limiting the number of dives, following recommendations provided by dive tables wherein limits are not met, and maintaining a diving profile that remains within the diving table guidelines have shown to reduce the likelihood of DCI in those with and without a PFO.[34]

TREATMENT: CURRENT RECOMMENDATIONS

Resuscitation as per standard guidelines should be performed as needed. First-line supportive management includes proper positioning of the diver to maintain airway, administration of oxygen, and intravenous fluid administration.[46] Management of DCI is outlined in **Fig. 2**. To protect and maintain airway, the diver should be placed in a supine or recovery position. Standing may cause further neurologic harm as bubbles travel along a gravity gradient.[47] Oxygen administration at the highest possible fraction of inspired oxygen is a Class 1C recommendation for DCI or arterial gas

Table 1
Summary of studies on patent foramen ovale closure in patients with decompression illness

Study, Year	Methodology	Study Size (n)	Follow-up	Results	Complications
Honek et al,[39] 2020	Prospective registry comparing the incidence of recurrent unprovoked DCI in catheter-based PFO closure group vs patients with grade 3 PFO practicing conservative diving practices	55 in the PFO closure group vs 98 in the conservative group	Mean (SD): 7.1 (3.8) y	Incidence of DCI: none in the PFO closure group vs 11% in the conservative group (P = .012)	Minor bleeding: 2 patients in the PFO closure group No major complications
Henzel et al,[43] 2018	Single-center experience evaluating recurrent DCI after transcatheter PFO closure in patients with history of DCI	11	Median (IQR): 91 (9–172) mo	No episodes of recurrent DCI at a mean maximum depth of 93.8 ± 35.6 m	No major complications
Koopsen et al,[11] 2018	Retrospective study evaluating recurrent DCI in patients with history of DCI referred to a cardiologist	29 patients with PFO, 6 with ASD, 27 patients with no PFO	Mean: 6.8 y	No recurrence of major DCS in either group	No major complications
Pearmen et al,[44] 2015	Retrospective audit of eligible divers who underwent PFO closure for prevention of DCI	105	—	2 divers with residual shunt required a second procedure 81/95 divers with follow-up bubble contrast echocardiography returned to unrestrictive diving	Atrial fibrillation: 2 patients Stroke: 1 patient in whom stroke was thought to be unrelated to the PFO closure

(continued on next page)

Table 1
(continued)

Study, Year	Methodology	Study Size (n)	Follow-up	Results	Complications
Honek et al,[40] 2014	Case-control study evaluating arterial bubbles by TCD under simulated diving conditions in catheter-based PFO closure group vs unrepaired high-grade PFO group	20 in the PFO closure group vs 27 in the conservative group	Median (IQR) time between PFO closure and simulated dive: 36 (17–81) mo	Incidence of arterial bubbles on TCD: 18-m dive: none in the PFO closure group vs 32% in the conservative group (P = .02) 50 m dive: none in the PFO closure group vs 88% in the conservative group (P<.01)	Minor bleeding: bleeding at puncture site with no need for intervention in PFO closure group No major complications
Billinger et al,[45] 2011	Prospective, nonrandomized, longitudinal study evaluating neurologic DCI in patients with a history of major DCI. Comparative groups: PFO with closure vs PFO without closure vs no PFO group	25 in PFO with closure vs 30 in PFO without closure vs 28 with no PFO	Mean (SD): 5.3 (0.3) y	Incidence of major neurologic DCI per 10,000 dives: 0.5 in the PFO closure group vs 35.8 in the PFO without closure group vs 0 in the no PFO group (P = .045) Incidence of ischemic brain lesions per 10,000 dives: 6 in the PFO closure group vs 104 in the PFO without closure group vs 16 in the no PFO group (P = .039)	No major complications

Abbreviations: ASD, atrial septal defect; DCI, decompression illness; IQR, interquartile range; PFO, patent foramen ovale; SD, standard deviation; TCD, transcranial Doppler.

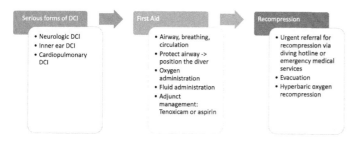

Fig. 2. Stepwise management of decompression illness.

embolism (without significant inert gas load) as per the latest Undersea and Hyperbaric Medical Society guidelines released in 2002.[48] Oxygen can be safely administered for up to 12 hours with air breaks. Administration beyond 12 hours is left to the treating physician's discretion. Oxygen helps lower the likelihood of requiring multiple recompressions and has been found to improve symptoms.[49] Administration of intravenous fluids, with either lactated Ringer solution or other dextrose-free isotonic fluid, is recommended as prolonged immersion can induce diuresis.[48] Hydration is essential as hemoconcentration and shock can be deadly manifestations of severe DCI. If fully conscious, noncaffeinated, nonalcoholic, and noncarbonated fluids containing sodium should be consumed. Water is an acceptable alternative.

Recompression with Hyperbaric Oxygen

Despite the lack of high-quality evidence, the definitive treatment of DCI is recompression in a hyperbaric chamber initially with 2.8-atm absolute (ATA) oxygen recompression.[5] Recompression therapy tables with US Navy Treatment Table 6 or Heliox (mixture of oxygen and helium) should be used for the initial management of DCI as they facilitate reduction in bubble size with pressure.[50] The recompression protocol can be either repeated or prolonged if response is poor with the initial session. After completion of initial treatment, in divers with residual symptoms, once-daily hyperbaric chamber treatment with 2.0 to 2.8-ATA oxygen recompression is used.[5] Hyperbaric oxygen facilitates reentry of bubbles from tissues into the vasculature and redistribution of bubbles within the blood vessels, allowing for gradual decompression. In a randomized trial of 180 divers with DCI who underwent hyperbaric oxygen treatment, a 7 day course of tenoxicam 20 mg in addition to hyperbaric oxygen was associated with a significant reduction in the number of hyperbaric oxygen sessions required for discharge.[51] Considering the limited size of the study population and no other clinical studies evaluating this, there are insufficient data to support

the use of tenoxicam as a part of the hyperbaric oxygen treatment protocol. In cases with no nearby facility with a hyperbaric chamber, in-water recompression at shallow depths of around 10 m can serve as an alternative.[5] However, the safety and efficacy of this approach is not established, with concerns for serious complications such as hypothermia, oxygen toxicity, seizure, and unconsciousness underwater.[5]

SUPPORTIVE MANAGEMENT

Adjunct management with aspirin or tenoxicam, a nonsteroidal anti-inflammatory drug (NSAID), which is a nonselective inhibitor of cyclooxygenase is a Class IIB, level C recommendation for the management of pain accompanying DCI according to the Undersea and Hyperbaric Medical Society guidelines.[48] In a placebo-controlled randomized trial consisting primarily of mild cases of DCI, tenoxicam was found to reduce the number of recompressions needed to achieve complete symptom resolution or a state of no further improvement.[51] Other NSAIDs are currently not recommended. Routine use of therapeutic anticoagulation or thrombolytics is not recommended in patients with neurologic DCI due to the risk of hemorrhage, particularly in inner ear or spinal cord DCI. In patients with neurologic DCI with leg weakness, enoxaparin injected subcutaneously should be used for routine deep venous thrombosis prophylaxis.[46] It is important to note that the above guideline recommendations have been extrapolated from findings in patients with traumatic spinal cord injury.[48] These medications or approaches have not been studied for safety and efficacy in patients with neurologic DCI.[48] Medications such as corticosteroids or lidocaine (for its antiarrhythmic effect) should not be used preemptively in anticipation of complications.[52]

FUTURE DIRECTIONS

Current evidence on the optimal management of DCI, particularly in the setting of PFO for secondary prevention of paradoxic embolism, is inadequate in quality and quantity. Although studies investigating the efficacy of percutaneous PFO closure in DCI have been conducted, large, randomized studies evaluating long-term outcomes in patients who continue to dive after the closure are required. Also, a "safe" diving depth for patients with history of DCI has been suggested based on the findings of small observational studies. Larger studies validating these findings are required. It has been more than a decade since the last revision to the best practice guidelines on the management of DCI was released by the Undersea and Hyperbaric Medical Society.[53] Presumably, this could be due to the lack of new studies with high-quality evidence. Additionally, adjunctive management of DCI requires in-depth and focused research as several of the recommendations are extrapolated from findings in traumatic brain injury patients. This again reflects the paucity of research in diving medicine.

CLINICS CARE POINTS

- Presence of PFO, particularly if high grade, increases the risk of DCI and its severe forms. However, routine screening for PFO is not recommended.

- In unprovoked or recurrent DCI, neurologic, cutaneous, or cardiopulmonary DCI, testing for PFO is indicated with bubble contrast echocardiography or TCD using provocative maneuvers.

- In patients with PFO and history of DCI, evaluation by a cardiologist with expertise in diving medicine is recommended.

- Consideration should be given to PFO closure if cessation of diving or conservative diving cannot be achieved.

- Prospective studies evaluating long-term outcomes in patients who continue to dive after PFO closure are required.

DISCLOSURE

The authors have nothing to disclose.

REFERENCES

1. Peppas S, Palaiodimos L, Nagraj S, et al. Right-to-Left shunt in divers with neurological decompression sickness: a systematic review and meta-analysis. Healthcare (Basel) 2023;11(10). https://doi.org/10.3390/healthcare11101407.

2. Palaiodimos L, Mahato P, Gershon A, et al. Chapter 13 - less recognized conditions associated with PFO: decompression illness, carcinoid heart disease, coronary spasm. In: Mojadidi MK, Meier B, Tobis JM, editors. Patent foramen ovale closure for stroke, myocardial infarction, peripheral embolism, migraine, and hypoxemia. Academic Press; 2020. p. 155–67.

3. Dardeau MR, Pollock NW, McDonald CM, et al. The incidence of decompression illness in 10 years of scientific diving. Diving Hyperb Med 2012;42(4): 195–200.

4. Honěk J, Šrámek M, Šefc L, et al. High-grade patent foramen ovale is a risk factor of unprovoked decompression sickness in recreational divers. J Cardiol 2019;74(6):519–23.

5. Mitchell SJ, Bennett MH, Moon RE. Decompression sickness and arterial gas embolism. N Engl J Med 2022;386(13):1254–64.

6. Torti SR, Billinger M, Schwerzmann M, et al. Risk of decompression illness among 230 divers in relation to the presence and size of patent foramen ovale. Eur Heart J 2004;25(12):1014–20.

7. Giblett JP, Williams LK, Kyranis S, et al. Patent foramen ovale closure: state of the Art. Interv Cardiol 2020;15:e15.

8. Fell SD. Available at: https://www.emedicinehealth.com/decompression_syndromes_the_bends/article_em.htm, (Accessed 2 October, 2023), 2023.

9. Hartig F, Reider N, Sojer M, et al. Livedo Racemosa - the pathophysiology of decompression-associated cutis marmorata and right/left shunt. Front Physiol 2020;11:994.

10. Xu W, Liu W, Huang G, et al. Decompression illness: clinical aspects of 5278 consecutive cases treated in a single hyperbaric unit. PLoS One 2012;7(11): e50079.

11. Koopsen R, Stella PR, Thijs KM, et al. Persistent foramen ovale closure in divers with a history of decompression sickness. Neth Heart J 2018; 26(11):535–9.

12. Strauss RS. Skin Bends: a cutaneous manifestation of decompression sickness. J Gen Intern Med 2019;34(10):2290.

13. Cantais E, Louge P, Suppini A, et al. Right-to-left shunt and risk of decompression illness with cochleovestibular and cerebral symptoms in divers: case control study in 101 consecutive dive accidents. Crit Care Med 2003;31(1):84–8.

14. Schwerzmann M, Seiler C, Lipp E, et al. Relation between directly detected patent foramen ovale and ischemic brain lesions in sport divers. Ann Intern Med 2001;134(1):21–4.

15. Balestra C, Germonpré P. Correlation between patent foramen ovale, cerebral "lesions" and Neuropsychometric testing in experienced sports divers: does diving damage the brain? Front Psychol 2016;7:696.

16. Boyd KL WA. Inner ear decompression sickness. StatPearls; 2024.

17. Vann RD, Butler FK, Mitchell SJ, et al. Decompression illness. Lancet 2011;377(9760):153–64.

18. Louka AM, Nagraj S, Adamou AT, et al. Risk Stratification Tools to guide a Personalized approach for cardiac Monitoring in embolic stroke of Undetermined Source. J Am Heart Assoc 2023;12(18): e030479.

19. Decompression illness in divers with or without patent foramen ovale. Ann Intern Med 2023;176(7): 934–9.

20. Favilla CG, Messé SR. Patent foramen ovale and stroke: current evidence and treatment options. Curr Opin Neurol 2020;33(1):10–6.

21. Palaiodimos L, Kokkinidis DG, Faillace RT, et al. Percutaneous closure of patent foramen ovale vs. medical treatment for patients with history of cryptogenic stroke: a systematic review and meta-analysis of randomized controlled trials. Cardiovasc Revasc Med 2018;19(7 Pt B):852–8.

22. Cartoni D, De Castro S, Valente G, et al. Identification of professional scuba divers with patent foramen ovale at risk for decompression illness. Am J Cardiol 2004;94(2):270–3.

23. Wilmshurst PT, Morrison WL, Walsh KP. Comparison of the size of persistent foramen ovale and atrial septal defects in divers with shunt-related decompression illness and in the general population. Diving Hyperb Med 2015;45(2):89–93.

24. Gempp E, Louge P, Blatteau JE, et al. Risks factors for recurrent neurological decompression sickness in recreational divers: a case-control study. J Sports Med Phys Fitness 2012;52(5):530–6.

25. Marabotti C, Scalzini A, Menicucci D, et al. Cardiovascular changes during SCUBA diving: an underwater Doppler echocardiographic study. Acta Physiol 2013;209(1):62–8.

26. Honĕk J, Šefc L, Honĕk T, et al. Patent foramen ovale in recreational and professional divers: an important and largely Unrecognized Problem. Can J Cardiol 2015;31(8):1061–6.

27. Erdem I, Yildiz S, Uzun G, et al. Cerebral white-matter lesions in asymptomatic military divers. Aviat Space Environ Med 2009;80(1):2–4.

28. Gempp E, Sbardella F, Stephant E, et al. Brain MRI signal abnormalities and right-to-left shunting in asymptomatic military divers. Aviat Space Environ Med 2010;81(11):1008–12.

29. Gerriets T, Tetzlaff K, Hutzelmann A, et al. Association between right-to left shunts and brain lesions in sport divers. Aviat Space Environ Med 2003; 74(10):1058–60.

30. Koch AE, Kampen J, Tetzlaff K, et al. Incidence of abnormal cerebral findings in the MRI of clinically healthy divers: role of a patent foramen ovale. Undersea Hyperb Med 2004;31(2):261–8.

31. Knauth M, Ries S, Pohimann S, et al. Cohort study of multiple brain lesions in sport divers: role of a patent foramen ovale. Bmj 1997;314(7082):701–5.

32. National Oceanic and Atmospheric Administration diving medical standards and procedures manual. National Oceanic and Atmospheric Administration diving medical standards and procedures manual. 2023. Available at: https://www.omao.noaa.gov/ sites/default/files/documents/Diving%20Medical% 20Standards%20and%20Procedures%20Manual% 2C%202010.pdf (Accessed 6 October, 2023).

33. Medical examination and assessment of working divers Health and Safety Executive. 2023. Available at: https://www.hse.gov.uk/pubns/ma1.pdf (Accessed 6 October, 2023).

34. Sykes O, Clark JE. Patent foramen ovale and scuba diving: a practical guide for physicians on when to refer for screening. Extrem Physiol Med 2013;2(1):10.

35. Pinto FJ. When and how to diagnose patent foramen ovale. Heart 2005;91(4):438–40.

36. Zito C, Dattilo G, Oreto G, et al. Patent foramen ovale: comparison among diagnostic strategies in cryptogenic stroke and migraine. Echocardiography 2009;26(5):495–503.

37. Katsanos AH, Psaltopoulou T, Sergentanis TN, et al. Transcranial Doppler versus transthoracic echocardiography for the detection of patent foramen ovale in patients with cryptogenic cerebral ischemia: a systematic review and diagnostic test accuracy meta-analysis. Ann Neurol 2016;79(4):625–35.

38. Percutaneous closure of patent foramen ovale for the secondary prevention of recurrent paradoxical embolism in divers. National Institute for Health and Care Excellence. Updated 2010, Available at: https://www.nice.org.uk/guidance/ipg371/chapter/ 2-The-procedure. (Accessed 6 October, 2023), 2023.

39. Honĕk J, Šrámek M, Honĕk T, et al. Patent foramen ovale closure is effective in divers: long-term results from the DIVE-PFO registry. J Am Coll Cardiol 2020; 76(9):1149–50.

40. Honĕk J, Šrámek M, Šefc L, et al. Effect of catheter-based patent foramen ovale closure on the occurrence of arterial bubbles in scuba divers. JACC Cardiovasc Interv 2014;7(4):403–8.

41. Abdelfattah OM, Sayed A, Elgendy IY, et al. Patent foramen ovale closure and decompression sickness among divers. Cardiovasc Revascularization Med 2022;40:160–2.

42. Smart D, Mitchell S, Wilmshurst P, et al. Joint position statement on persistent foramen ovale (PFO) and diving. South Pacific underwater medicine Society (SPUMS) and the United Kingdom sports diving medical Committee (UKSDMC). Diving Hyperb Med 2015;45(2):129–31.

43. Henzel J, Rudziński PN, Kłopotowski M, et al. Transcatheter closure of patent foramen ovale for the

secondary prevention of decompression illness in professional divers: a single-centre experience with long-term follow-up. Kardiol Pol 2018;76(1): 153–7.

44. Pearman A, Bugeja L, Nelson M, et al. An audit of persistent foramen ovale closure in 105 divers. Diving Hyperb Med 2015;45(2):94–7.

45. Michael B, Rainer Z, Raffaela M, et al. Patent foramen ovale closure in recreational divers: effect on decompression illness and ischaemic brain lesions during long-term follow-up. Heart 2011;97(23):1932.

46. Richard E. and Moon S.M., Hyperbaric treatment for decompression sickness: current recommendations, Available at: https://dukespace.lib.duke.edu/dspace/bitstream/handle/10161/23433/Moon%20Hyperbaric%20treatment%20for%20decompression%20sickness-current%20recommendations%20Undersea%20Hyperb%20Med%202019.pdf?sequence=2&isAllowed=y, (Accessed 8 October, 2023), 2019.

47. Banham ND, Saw J, Hankey GJ, et al. Cerebral arterial gas embolism proven by computed tomography following transthoracic echocardiography using bubble contrast. Diving Hyperb Med 2020;50(3): 300–2.

48. Adjunctive therapy for decompression illness (DCI): summary of undersea and hyperbaric medical society guidelines. Undersea and hyperbaric medical society, Available at: https://www.uhms.org/images/Position-Statements/adjunctive_committee_summary.pdf (Accessed 8 October, 2023), 2023.

49. Longphre JM, Denoble PJ, Moon RE, et al. First aid normobaric oxygen for the treatment of recreational diving injuries. Undersea Hyperb Med 2007;34(1): 43–9.

50. Mathieu D, Marroni A, Kot J. Tenth European Consensus Conference on Hyperbaric Medicine: recommendations for accepted and non-accepted clinical indications and practice of hyperbaric oxygen treatment. Diving Hyperb Med 2017;47(1): 24–32.

51. Bennett M, Mitchell S, Dominguez A. Adjunctive treatment of decompression illness with a non-steroidal anti-inflammatory drug (tenoxicam) reduces compression requirement. Undersea Hyperb Med 2003;30(3):195–205.

52. Habibi MR, Habibi V, Habibi A, et al. Lidocaine dose-response effect on postoperative cognitive deficit: meta-analysis and meta-regression. Expert Rev Clin Pharmacol 2018;11(4):361–71.

53. UHMS Best Practice Guidelines Prevention and Treatment of Decompression Sickness and Arterial Gas Embolism, Available at: https://www.uhms.org/images/DCS-AGE-Committee/dcsandage_prevandmgt_uhms-fi.pdf. UHMS Best Practice Guidelines. (Accessed 28 October, 2023), 2023.

Practical Aspects of Patent Foramen Ovale Closure
Ultrasound and Fluoroscopic Guidance

Kerstin Piayda, MD, MSc[a,b], Stefan Bertog, MD[a,c], Mackenzie Mbai, MD[c], Alok Sharma, MD[c], Verena Veulemans, MD[d], Horst Sievert, MD[a,*]

KEYWORDS

- PFO closure • Periprocedural management • TEE • ICE • Angiographic guidance
- Fluoroscopic guidance

KEY POINTS

- Percutaneous persistend foramen ovale (PFO) closure has become a well-established method to mitigate paradoxic embolism in a carefully selected group of patients.
- Intraprocedural guidance for PFO closure can be performed in various ways, and each method has its advantages and disadvantages.
- Guidance by transesophageal echocardiography and fluoroscopy offers high-resolution two-dimesnional (2D)/three-dimensional (3D) imaging of the anatomy, the device, and surrounding structures. However, transesophageal echocardiography requires the presence of a peri-interventional imager and conscious sedation (or endotracheal intubation).
- Guidance by intracardiac echocardiography and fluoroscopy omits the need for conscious sedation (or endotracheal intubation) and can be performed by a single operator. However, vascular access site and bleeding complications, as well as the additional cost of the single-use intracardiac echo probes have to be taken into account.
- Guidance by fluoroscopy alone simplifies the procedure but may be associated with a higher rate of residual shunting and should be reserved for experienced operators and straightforward PFO anatomies.

 Video content accompanies this article at http://www.cardiology.theclinics.com.

INTRODUCTION

Percutaneous PFO closure has become a well-established method to prevent paradoxic embolism in a carefully selected group of patients.[1–3] Landmark trials[4–6] paved the way for integration of PFO closure into daily clinical practice. However, practical aspects including periprocedural guidance are less well examined, evolved over time, and profited from technical developments in the imaging field in the last decades. In general, the combination of an echocardiographic technique, either transesophageal echocardiography (TEE) or intracardiac echocardiography (ICE), in combination with fluoroscopy is a popular approach. Fluoroscopic guidance alone is also established, and a few centers work with transthoracic echocardiography (TTE) as a guiding tool.

a Cardiovascular Center Frankfurt, Frankfurt, Germany; b Department of Cardiology and Vascular Medicine, University Hospital Gießen and Marburg, Gießen, Germany; c Minneapolis Veterans Affairs Medical Center, Minneapolis, MN, USA; d Department of Cardiology, Pneumology and Vascular Medicine, University Hospital Düsseldorf, Düsseldorf, Germany
* Corresponding author. CardioVascularCenter (CVC) Frankfurt, Seckbacker Landstrasse 65, Frankfurt 60389, Germany.
E-mail address: horstsievertmd@aol.com

Cardiol Clin 42 (2024) 537–545
https://doi.org/10.1016/j.ccl.2024.02.001

An overview of important advantages and disadvantages of most commonly used image guidance tools during PFO closure is outlined in **Table 1**.

Independent of the imaging modality used during PFO closure, it is important to recognize that comparability of effective PFO closure is limited. The literature differentiates between effective PFO closure (ie, defined post hoc as freedom from a larger shunt[4]) and complete closure. However, there is no single, widely accepted grading scheme to quantify residual shunting after device placement. It also depends on how the bubble contrast is injected. Unselective injection (Video 1) is used in the majority of cases, but selective injections may have a higher sensitivity to reveal residual shunting (Video 2). Nonetheless, in some pivotal randomized trials demonstrating a stroke risk reduction with PFO closure, a residual shunt of less than 10 bubbles has been used to define effective closure, and when reported by the investigators, complete closure rates have typically been less than 90%, with effective closure rates between 90% and 100%. In the RESPECT trial (using Amplatzer PFO occluders), for example, the complete and effective closure rates were 73% and 94%, respectively in the 6 month echocardiographic follow-up.[5] In the REDUCE trial (using a Gore septal occluder or the Helex device), complete and effective closure rates were 76% and 99%.[4] Furthermore, the presence or absence of a residual shunt appears to be a dynamic phenomenon, with varying shunt rates over time. Some residual shunts diminish, especially within the first 12 months. However, it is not uncommon to find a residual shunt at later follow-up in cases where no shunt was seen previously. For example, in a study of patients who were determined to have no residual shunt at 6 months by intracranial Doppler, 29% were found to have a shunt at approximately 5 year follow-up.[7] Hence, it is likely that the complete closure rates reported in aforementioned pivotal trials are an overestimate because, once considered closed, echocardiographic follow-up was no longer required. In patients with moderate to large shunts, a long-term clinical and echocardiographic follow-up should be considered, since in some studies, residual shunting was associated with higher recurrent transient ischemic attack or stroke.[8]

GUIDANCE DURING PFO CLOSURE
Transthoracic Echocardiography with (or without) Fluoroscopy

Next to transcranial Doppler or TEE, TTE with bubble contrast is one of the most common first-line screening tools to detect a PFO. It has a sensitivity of 46%,[9] which can be improved to up to 90% with harmonic imaging,[10,11] but restricted ability to detect PFOs with a small right-to-left shunt.[9] In a limited fashion, TTE is also used for periprocedural guidance during PFO closure. TTE guidance has been performed with[12] and without fluoroscopy.[13] In the purely TTE-guided approach, the long-term closure rate was 90.4%, and the authors describe a lengthy learning curve because of the fundamentally different image display as compared to TEE.[13] Tracking of the catheter and guidewire crossing of the septum are less easy to monitor with transthoracic imaging. Additionally, unfavorable body habitus may limit the acoustic window. Hence, this approach should be reserved for experienced teams, straightforward PFO anatomies, and good imaging windows, especially in the apical and subcostal views.

2D/3D TRANSESOPHAGEAL ECHOCARDIOGRAPHY WITH (OR WITHOUT) FLUOROSCOPY

Fluoroscopy with echocardiographic guidance by TEE is an established way to perform PFO closure. This approach offers high-resolution, real-time 2D and 3D imaging of the device, the catheters, and the anatomy itself. Final device position and residual shunting can directly be evaluated. Disadvantages of this method include conscious sedation or general anesthesia because some patients placed in a supine position for the intervention do not tolerate TEE monitoring well. In addition, TEE (under conscious sedation) may be associated with a risk of aspiration and esophageal trauma.[14] In general, TEE-related adverse events during structural heart disease interventions are clinically relevant and increase with the complexity and duration of the procedure.[15] Uninterrupted TEE guidance for PFO closure may only be reserved for complex cases. Simplified approaches include a vastly fluoroscopy-guided approach with only a brisk TEE insertion just prior to device release for guidance during the most important procedural steps.[16] Nevertheless, TEE guidance requires additional support by an imaging specialist and this setup may increase the turnaround time in the catheter laboratory. TEE is semi-invasive and time-consuming. A recent meta-analysis, which compared TEE and ICE-guided closure of interatrial communications, showed that patients with an ICE-guided approach had a shorter fluoroscopy time, procedure duration, and a shorter length of in-hospital stay.[17] It should, however, be noted that this analysis was limited by selection bias because all included studies were cohort studies.

Table 1
Summary of advantages and disadvantages of most common imaging modalities during PFO closure

Fluoroscopy + TEE		Fluoroscopy + ICE		Fluoroscopy Alone	
Advantages	Disadvantages	Advantages	Disadvantages	Advantages	Disadvantages
High-resolution imaging of the interatrial septum (IAS) and surrounding structures	Requires additional support	Single operator, no echo support needed	May add additional costs (depending on jurisdiction)	Single operator, no echo support needed	Does not allow for high-resolution imaging
Widely available (if compared to ICE)	Usually requires anesthesia or sedation	Avoids anesthesia or sedation	Vascular complications	Avoids anesthesia or sedation	May be reserved for experienced operators and straight forward PFO anatomies
Superior image quality to TTE	Risk of esophageal trauma and aspiration	Comparable imaging quality to TEE	May cause pericardial perfusion or arrhythmias		
Device position and residual shunting can be evaluated	Patient discomfort	Patient comfort		Patient comfort	
		Shorter procedure duration and fluoroscopy times (if compared to TEE)			
		No risk for esophageal trauma or aspiration			

Recent developments in this field include the use of micro-TEE probes.[18] Miniaturization of ultrasound probes generally results in technical trade-offs with lower frame rates and decreased spatial resolution. Early generation microprobes allowed for 2D imaging, color Doppler, pulse-wave and continuous-wave Doppler, motion mode, and color flow motion-mode features. Image quality was lower as compared to conventional TEE probes but still rated sufficient for procedural guidance.[19] General Electric Health-Care and Phillips Healthcare now offer a probe with 3D imaging capacity. This probe may be primarily used in pediatric patients but can also be used in adults undergoing structural heart diseases interventions.[20] Further developments include technical improvements of the current ultrasound generation; deep learning algorithms are used to enhance lateral resolution in 3D imaging with adaptive beamforming.[21]

In practice, before vascular access is gained by the interventionalist, the imager can already assess the interatrial septal anatomy, morphology, and surrounding structures. Selected TEE views to guide PFO closure are displayed in **Fig. 1**. Other, potential sources of emboli should be visualized (ie, left atrial appendage, Eustachian valve, Chiari network, and intracardiac masses). To guide PFO closure, the probe is most commonly placed in a mid-esophageal position in the transverse plane at 0°, resembling a 4-chamber view, or in the so-called bi-caval view at 90° to 110° as well as the short axis view at 50° to 60°. The sector width and depth should be optimized to obtain a central view of the interatrial septum. Sometimes, rotating the imaging plane by 10° to 30° with simultaneous anticlockwise turning of the probe can improve visualization. Next to 2D biplane imaging, 3D imaging can give a comprehensive overview of the anatomy and can assist the interventionalist with wire crossing of the septum and other procedural steps. The total septum length should be measured and an appropriate device and device size should be selected. A prominent Eustachian valve may impede the placement of softer PFO devices, while a prominent Chiari network almost never causes interference.[22] Echocardiography tends to underestimate PFO size. Especially in patients with a complex anatomy (ie, aneurysmatic interatrial septum) (Video 3), balloon sizing (with the stop-flow technique) can be helpful to determine the true PFO size[23] (**Fig. 2**).

During the deployment process, the spatial relationship between the occluder, the septum, and surrounding structures is visualized. Before final device release, a wiggle test is performed, and the final device release is monitored. The imager should check for residual shunting and other procedure-related complications such as pericardial effusion.

Real-time fusion of dynamic images (ie, echocardiographic images are superimposed on angiography) can facilitate spatial orientation,[15] especially for learners or in patients with challenging anatomies.

Seldomly, a pure TEE-guided approach without fluoroscopy is used to guide PFO closure.[24,25] This method is completely radiation free and does not require contrast agent application.

2D/3D INTRACARDIAC ECHOCARDIOGRAPHY WITH (OR WITHOUT) FLUOROSCOPY

In contrast to TEE, ICE only has a role in peri-interventional imaging and is not used for pure diagnostic purposes. In recent years, it has emerged to an attractive alternative to TEE in the guidance of structural heart disease interventions.[26–29] In the United States, ICE-guided closure of interatrial communications increased from 9.7% (2003) to 50.6% (2014) in slightly more than a decade.[30]

TEE-specific complications like aspiration, esophageal trauma, or damage of the oral cavity are avoided. Patients with absolute or relative contraindications for TEE (ie, esophageal varices, cervical/thoracic spinal disease, and certain coagulopathies) can be treated with lower risk for procedure-related complications. During the intervention, ICE omits the need for conscious sedation or general anesthesia and hence improves patient comfort. It is single operator-dependent and no additional support by an imager is necessary. With the latter, staff cost, procedure duration,

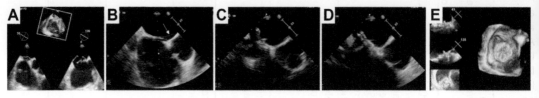

Fig. 1. Selected TEE views during PFO closure. (*A*) 3D view of the aneurysmatic interatrial septum with a prominent Eustachian valve. (*B*) Guide-wire crossing through the interatrial defect (*white arrow*). Development of the (*C*) left atrial and (*D*) right atrial disk under 2D guidance. (*E*) 3D assessment of the final PFO occluder position.

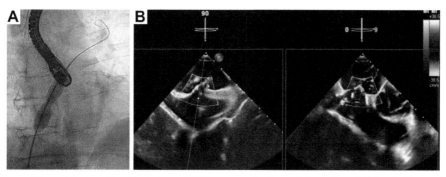

Fig. 2. Balloon sizing with stop-flow technique. (*A*) Fluoroscopic view of the inflated sizing balloon which shows a waist across the defect. (*B*) Transesophageal biplane imaging of the inflated balloon with color Doppler imaging. Once the balloon reaches the size of the defect, color flow over the defect stops, and the size of balloon is measured to indirectly determine PFO dimensions.

and turnaround times in the cath laboratory can be reduced but have to be weighed against the additional costs of the catheter,[31] which is a medical disposable. In Europe, the majority of health care systems do not reimburse ICE catheters, and additional costs remain with the hospital which is a significant drawback. In comparison, TEE machines and equipment are available in departments specialized on the treatment of structural heart disease anyway, and the salary of the imager is included in overhead costs. A cost analysis from the United States, which investigated the use of ICE during left atrial appendage occlusion, came to the conclusion that in an adjusted analysis, major complications rates were comparable between ICE and TEE, and intrahospital length of stay was similar. The ICE group had an excess cost of hospitalization, amounting to $ 1769 per case.[32] To our knowledge, no comprehensive, full economic evaluation has been performed so far with the inclusion of a different jurisdiction to investigate the cost-effectiveness of ICE guidance during structural heart disease interventions. Other potential disadvantages of ICE include, but are not limited to, higher time expenditure of the interventionalist, vascular access site complications and bleeding due to catheter sizes up to 12.5 French, arrhythmias, or intracardiac damage caused by the device itself or interference with other material. Early generation ICE catheters only allowed 2D imaging, further development steps included 3D rendering, and the latest generation of ICE probes allows real-time four-dimensional (4D) volume image acquisition with multiplanar reconstruction. Although ICE offers less temporal resolution and limited viewing depth as compared to TEE, the latter often allows only a suboptimal view on the lower part of the interatrial septum[33,34] as compared to ICE. A learning curve for the use of ICE is acknowledged[27,35] but has not been scientifically investigated. The steepness of the learning

curve potentially depends on the already acquired knowledge on standard TEE views for PFO closure since those are almost congruent with ICE views, and on the ability of handling, the ICE catheter itself. In case of PFO closure, a shorter procedure duration and radiation exposure were described,[31,36] while the use of ICE leads to less congruent results regarding radiation and contrast agent exposure during other structural heart disease interventions.[27] The use of ICE can be pre-scheduled in case of already preidentified challenging anatomies, or in case, nonconclusive or limited screening TEE images are available. It may also have its role as a "stand-by-tool," in case of difficult septal crossing or if other unforeseen difficulties arise during the procedure.[37] However, TEE monitoring under general anesthesia or conscious sedation is still a widely accepted alternative.

In practice, the procedure is performed with local anesthesia or conscious sedation. Two, single right venous accesses are established. To minimize interaction, most operators prefer to keep the ICE sheath access inferior to the PFO device access. Alternatively, the left femoral vein can be used for ICE access and the right for device access. Prior to any other device placement, the ICE catheter is advanced via the inferior vena cava to the right atrium. Advancement through a long sheath to avoid interference of the catheter with the pelvic veins may be preferable. The probe is then advanced to a neutral position in the mid-to-low right atrium, the so-called "home-view" (30° clockwise rotation and small anterior tilt of the probe). Here, important cardiac structures such as the tricuspid and aortic valve, the pulmonic valve in the right ventricular outflow tract can be visualized. Afterward, septal long-axis (through posterior tilting of the probe) and septal short-axis (through minimizing the clockwise rotation in combination with a slight left or right tilting of the probe) views are

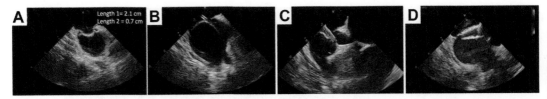

Fig. 3. Selected ICE views during PFO closure. (*A*) Initial assessment of the interatrial anatomy and morphology showing a hypermobile septum. (*B*) Guidance of defect crossing. (*C*) Monitoring of step-wise device deployment (in this case the left atrial disk is developed). (*D*) Final check for residual shunting with color Doppler flow.

mainly used to guide PFO closure. In the short- and long-axis view, the interatrial septum can be interrogated, wire crossing and advancement of the sheath and device visualized, and the full deployment process can be monitored (**Fig. 3**). In the end, comparable to TEE guidance, the device is assessed for correct and stable position ("tug/wiggle test," Video 4) as well as complete sealing. The ICE catheter is maneuvered back to the home position, allowing for a final sweep to rule out pericardial effusion. The device is removed and hemostasis may be achieved by a figure-of-8 suture with additional manual pressure or other closing methods of choice. Future applications may simplify the use of ICE: a machine learning-based algorithm facilitated the roll angle prediction for ICE catheter placements within the heart on the basis of landmark scalar values from biplane fluoroscopy images.[38]

FLUOROSCOPY GUIDANCE ALONE

First described in 2004, PFO closure can be performed under fluoroscopic guidance alone.[39] In principle, angiographic guidance alone may allow for shorter procedure duration, lower work force requirements, decreased costs and higher patient comfort. In addition, echocardiographic-related complications, such as aspiration, esophageal trauma, or vascular complications, in case of ICE, can be avoided.

Several studies[40–44] describe the feasibility and safety of this approach. Initial concerns of higher device malpositioning rates could not be proven. Residual shunts, which are a predictor for recurrent stroke,[8,45] were detected in up to 9%[42] of patients, whereas some echo-guided investigations showed complete shunt elimination rates of 98% and 99%,[46,47] although the definition of incomplete closure varies from study to study. In a propensity-matched comparison between an echo-guided and a pure fluoroscopy-guided approach, the latter had higher re-intervention rates due to incomplete closure during follow-up.[48] However, those findings might lack generalizability. In a head-to-head comparison, procedure duration and fluoroscopy time were lower in the angiographic guidance alone group as compared to TEE or ICE.[44] Hildick-Smith and colleagues[49] tested a "stand-by echo approach." In 9% of patients, the conversion from fluoroscopic guidance alone to ICE-controlled PFO closure was necessary, due to larger size defects (>15 mm), difficulties of crossing the interatrial septum or a long tunnel requiring transseptal puncture for successful device deployment. In other studies, the

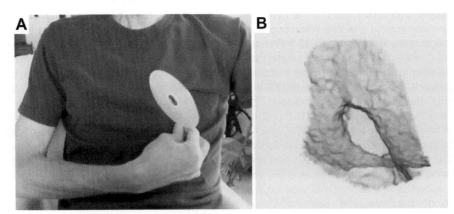

Fig. 4. Anatomical orientation of the interatrial septum. (*A*) Simulation of the interatrial septum position within the body to illustrate why left anterior and oblique (LAO) cranial (40°/40°) view can be helpful to identify the PFO position during the procedure. (*B*) Computed tomography-derived simulation of the interatrial septum.

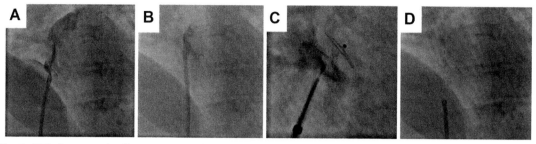

Fig. 5. PFO closure under fluoroscopic guidance alone. (*A*) Hand injection of contrast medium after wire crossing of the interatrial septum through the catheter (*B*) development of the left and (*C*) right atrial disc (*D*) final device position.

conversion rate to an echocardiographic supported approach remained lower[44] or the use of echocardiography was not necessary.[42]

Pure fluoroscopy guidance may be reserved for experienced operators and straightforward PFO anatomies (ie, small defects, short PFO tunnel length, and single septum fenestration).

In practice, right atrial angiography through a pigtail catheter in the left anterior and oblique cranial (40°/40°) view using power injection of contrast can help identify the PFO position since the septum is portrayed "enface" (**Fig. 4**). It is helpful to allow enough fluoroscopic time for the contrast to appear in the left atrium for better visualization and understanding of the anatomy. Hand injection of contrast agent through the catheter may allow the entry point identification of the tunnel. However, frequently the use of a power injector is needed. If the PFO is not easily identified, patients can be instructed to perform Valsalva maneuvers after contrast injection. The so-called "Pacman sign"[50] refers to the fluoroscopic picture of the deployed device in an orthogonal view, which should be achieved before final release to ensure proper device deployment: the cranial parts of both the left and the right atrial disk should resemble open jaws biting into the septum secundum. **Fig. 5** illustrates the important procedural steps of PFO closure with fluoroscopic guidance alone.

Newer generation technologies, such as the suture-mediated, deviceless NobleStitch EL (Heartstitch, Inc, Fountain Valley, CA), entirely rely on fluoroscopic guidance only and do not require any echocardiographic support.

SUMMARY AND KEY LEARNING POINTS

Interventional PFO closure has emerged to a safe and effective treatment option in well-selected patients to avoid the future risk of stroke. The procedure can be guided by fluoroscopy alone or can additionally be supported by TTE, TEE, or ICE. Each modality has its own advantages and disadvantages. Sometimes conversion from a fluoroscopy alone to an echo-guided approach is necessary to ensure procedural success. Depending on experience, availability, patient anatomy, and device choice, a case-based decision should be made to ensure best clinical results and patient safety.

CLINICS CARE POINTS

- If PFO closure is performed by transesophageal guidance (and fluoroscopy), be aware that this technique requires conscious sedation (or endotracheal intubation) and may be associated with esophageal trauma.

- In case PFO closure is guided by intracardiac echocardiography, be aware of potential bleeding complications and vascular access site complications.

- If PFO closure is guided by fluoroscopy alone, be aware of higher residual shunting rates during follow-up. This technique should be reserved for experienced operators and straightforward PFO anatomies.

DISCLOSURE

H. Sievert has received study honoraria to institution, travel expenses and consulting fees from 4tech Cardio, Abbott, Ablative Solutions, Adona Medical, Akura Medical, Ancora Heart, Append Medical, Axon, Bavaria Medizin Technologie GmbH, Bioventrix, Boston Scientific, Cardiac Dimensions, Cardiac Success, Cardimed, Cardionovum, Celonova, Contego, Coramaze, Croivalve, CSL Behring LLC, CVRx, Dinova, Edwards, Endobar, Endologix, Endomatic, Esperion Therapeutics, Inc, Hangzhou Nuomao Medtech, Holistick Medical, Intershunt, Intervene, K2, Laminar, Lifetech, Magenta, Maquet Getinge Group,

Metavention, Mitralix, Mokita, Neurotronic, NXT Biomedical, Occlutech, Recor, Renal Guard, Shifamed, Terumo, Trisol, Vascular Dynamics, Vectorious Medtech, Venus, Venock, Vivasure Medical, Vvital Biomed, and Whiteswell.

SUPPLEMENTARY DATA

Supplementary data related to this article can be found online at https://doi.org/10.1016/j.ccl.2024.02.001.

REFERENCES

1. Pristipino C, Sievert H, D'Ascenzo F, et al. European position paper on the management of patients with patent foramen ovale. General approach and left circulation thromboembolism. Eur Heart J 2019;40(38):3182–95.
2. Singh V, Badheka AO, Patel NJ, et al. Influence of hospital volume on outcomes of percutaneous atrial septal defect and patent foramen ovale closure: a 10-years US perspective. Catheter Cardiovasc Interv 2015;85(6):1073–81.
3. Collado FMS, Poulin MF, Murphy JJ, et al. Patent foramen ovale closure for stroke prevention and other disorders. J Am Heart Assoc 2018;7(12).
4. Sondergaard L, Kasner SE, Rhodes JF, et al. Patent foramen ovale closure or antiplatelet therapy for cryptogenic stroke. N Engl J Med 2017;377(11):1033–42.
5. Carroll JD, Saver JL, Thaler DE, et al. Closure of patent foramen ovale versus medical therapy after cryptogenic stroke. N Engl J Med 2013;368(12):1092–100.
6. Saver JL, Carroll JD, Thaler DE, et al. Long-term outcomes of patent foramen ovale closure or medical therapy after stroke. N Engl J Med 2017;377(11):1022–32.
7. Cheli M, Canepa M, Brunelli C, et al. Recurrent and residual shunts after patent foramen ovale closure: results from a long-term transcranial Doppler study. J Intervent Cardiol 2015;28(6):600–8.
8. Deng W, Yin S, McMullin D, et al. Residual shunt after patent foramen ovale closure and long-term stroke recurrence: a prospective cohort study. Ann Intern Med 2020;172(11):717–25.
9. Ren P, Li K, Lu X, et al. Diagnostic value of transthoracic echocardiography for patent foramen ovale: a meta-analysis. Ultrasound Med Biol 2013;39(10):1743–50.
10. Madala D, Zaroff JG, Hourigan L, et al. Harmonic imaging improves sensitivity at the expense of specificity in the detection of patent foramen ovale. Echocardiography 2004;21(1):33–6.
11. Mojadidi MK, Winoker JS, Roberts SC, et al. Two-dimensional echocardiography using second harmonic imaging for the diagnosis of intracardiac right-to-left shunt: a meta-analysis of prospective studies. Int J Cardiovasc Imag 2014;30(5):911–23.
12. Oto A, Aytemir K, Ozkutlu S, et al. Transthoracic echocardiography guidance during percutaneous closure of patent foramen ovale. Echocardiography 2011;28(10):1074–80.
13. Yang T, Butera G, Ou-Yang WB, et al. Percutaneous closure of patent foramen ovale under transthoracic echocardiography guidance-midterm results. J Thorac Dis 2019;11(6):2297–304.
14. Freitas-Ferraz AB, Bernier M, Vaillancourt R, et al. Safety of transesophageal echocardiography to guide structural cardiac interventions. J Am Coll Cardiol 2020;75(25):3164–73.
15. Afzal S, Zeus T, Hofsahs T, et al. Safety of transoesophageal echocardiography during structural heart disease interventions under procedural sedation: a single-centre study. Eur Heart J Cardiovasc Imaging 2022;24(1):68–77.
16. Achim A, Hochegger P, Kanoun Schnur SS, et al. Transesophageal echocardiography-guided versus fluoroscopy-guided patent foramen ovale closure: a single center registry. Echocardiography 2023;40(7):657–63.
17. Lan Q, Wu F, Ye X, et al. Intracardiac vs. transesophageal echocardiography for guiding transcatheter closure of interatrial communications: a systematic review and meta-analysis. Front Cardiovasc Med 2023;10:1082663.
18. Snijder RJR, Renes LE, Swaans MJ, et al. Microtransesophageal echocardiographic guidance during percutaneous interatrial septal closure without general anaesthesia. J Intervent Cardiol 2020;2020:1462140.
19. Nijenhuis VJ, Alipour A, Wunderlich NC, et al. Feasibility of multiplane microtransoesophageal echocardiographic guidance in structural heart disease transcatheter interventions in adults. Neth Heart J 2017;25(12):669–74.
20. 9VT -D. The world's first mini 3D TEE probe [press release]. GE HealthCare 2023;17:2023.
21. Ossenkoppele BW, Luijten B, Bera D, et al. Improving lateral resolution in 3-D imaging with micro-beamforming through adaptive beamforming by deep learning. Ultrasound Med Biol 2023;49(1):237–55.
22. Davison P, Clift PF, Steeds RP. The role of echocardiography in diagnosis, monitoring closure and post-procedural assessment of patent foramen ovale. Eur J Echocardiogr 2010;11(10):i27–34.
23. Kumar P, Rusheen J, Tobis JM. A comparison of methods to determine patent foramen ovale size. Catheter Cardiovasc Interv 2020;96(6):E621–9.
24. Wang S, Zhu G, Liu Z, et al. Only transesophageal echocardiography guided patent foramen ovale closure: a single-center experience. Front Surg 2022;9:977959.

25. Han Y, Zhang X, Zhang F. Patent foramen ovale closure by using transesophageal echocardiography for cryptogenic stroke: single center experience in 132 consecutive patients. J Cardiothorac Surg 2020;15(1):11.

26. Mullen MJ, Dias BF, Walker F, et al. Intracardiac echocardiography guided device closure of atrial septal defects. J Am Coll Cardiol 2003;41(2):285–92.

27. Nielsen-Kudsk JE, Berti S, Caprioglio F, et al. Intracardiac echocardiography to guide watchman FLX implantation: the ICE LAA study. JACC Cardiovasc Interv 2023;16(6):643–51.

28. Ruparelia N, Cao J, Newton JD, et al. Paravalvular leak closure under intracardiac echocardiographic guidance. Catheter Cardiovasc Interv 2018;91(5):958–65.

29. Akkaya E, Vuruskan E, Zorlu A, et al. Aortic intracardiac echocardiography-guided septal puncture during mitral valvuloplasty. Eur Heart J Cardiovasc Imaging 2014;15(1):70–6.

30. Alqahtani F, Bhirud A, Aljohani S, et al. Intracardiac versus transesophageal echocardiography to guide transcatheter closure of interatrial communications: nationwide trend and comparative analysis. J Intervent Cardiol 2017;30(3):234–41.

31. Bartel T, Konorza T, Arjumand J, et al. Intracardiac echocardiography is superior to conventional monitoring for guiding device closure of interatrial communications. Circulation 2003;107(6):795–7.

32. Zahid S, Gowda S, Hashem A, et al. Feasibility and safety of intracardiac echocardiography use in transcatheter left atrial appendage closure procedures. J Soc Cardiovascul Angiograph Interven 2022;1(6):100510.

33. Hijazi Z, Wang Z, Cao Q, et al. Transcatheter closure of atrial septal defects and patent foramen ovale under intracardiac echocardiographic guidance: feasibility and comparison with transesophageal echocardiography. Catheter Cardiovasc Interv 2001;52(2):194–9.

34. Koenig P, Cao QL. Echocardiographic guidance of transcatheter closure of atrial septal defects: is intracardiac echocardiography better than transesophageal echocardiography? Pediatr Cardiol 2005;26(2):135–9.

35. Alkhouli M, Hijazi ZM, Holmes DR Jr, et al. Intracardiac echocardiography in structural heart disease interventions. JACC Cardiovasc Interv 2018;11(21):2133–47.

36. Bartel T, Konorza T, Neudorf U, et al. Intracardiac echocardiography: an ideal guiding tool for device closure of interatrial communications. Eur J Echocardiogr 2005;6(2):92–6.

37. Barker M, Muthuppalaniappan AM, Abrahamyan L, et al. Periprocedural outcomes of fluoroscopy-guided patent foramen ovale closure with selective use of intracardiac echocardiography. Can J Cardiol 2020;36(10):1608–15.

38. Annabestani M, Caprio A, Wong SC, et al. A machine learning-based roll angle prediction for intracardiac echocardiography catheter during Bi-plane fluoroscopy. Appl Sci 2023;13(6):3483.

39. Varma C, Benson LN, Warr MR, et al. Clinical outcomes of patent foramen ovale closure for paradoxical emboli without echocardiographic guidance. Catheter Cardiovasc Interv 2004;62(4):519–25.

40. Jamshidi P, Wahl A, Windecker S, et al. Percutaneous closure of patent foramen ovale without echocardiographic guidance. Indian Heart J 2007;59(6):459–62.

41. Fateh-Moghadam S, Steeg M, Dietz R, et al. Is routine ultrasound guidance really necessary for closure of patent foramen ovale using the Amplatzer PFO occluder? Catheter Cardiovasc Interv 2009;73(3):361–6.

42. Wahl A, Tai T, Praz F, et al. Late results after percutaneous closure of patent foramen ovale for secondary prevention of paradoxical embolism using the amplatzer PFO occluder without intraprocedural echocardiography: effect of device size. JACC Cardiovasc Interv 2009;2(2):116–23.

43. Siddiqui IF, Michaels AD. Percutaneous patent foramen ovale closure using Helex and Amplatzer devices without intraprocedural echocardiographic guidance. J Intervent Cardiol 2011;24(3):271–7.

44. Mangieri A, Godino C, Montorfano M, et al. PFO closure with only fluoroscopic guidance: 7 years real-world single centre experience. Catheter Cardiovasc Interv 2015;86(1):105–12.

45. Wahl A, Krumsdorf U, Meier B, et al. Transcatheter treatment of atrial septal aneurysm associated with patent foramen ovale for prevention of recurrent paradoxical embolism in high-risk patients. J Am Coll Cardiol 2005;45(3):377–80.

46. Onorato E, Melzi G, Casilli F, et al. Patent foramen ovale with paradoxical embolism: mid-term results of transcatheter closure in 256 patients. J Intervent Cardiol 2003;16(1):43–50.

47. Martin F, Sanchez PL, Doherty E, et al. Percutaneous transcatheter closure of patent foramen ovale in patients with paradoxical embolism. Circulation 2002;106(9):1121–6.

48. Scacciatella P, Meynet I, Giorgi M, et al. Angiography vs transesophageal echocardiography-guided patent foramen ovale closure: a propensity score matched analysis of a two-center registry. Echocardiography 2018;35(6):834–40.

49. Hildick-Smith D, Behan M, Haworth P, et al. Patent foramen ovale closure without echocardiographic control: use of "standby" intracardiac ultrasound. JACC Cardiovasc Interv 2008;1(4):387–91.

50. Meier B. Pacman sign during device closure of the patent foramen ovale. Catheter Cardiovasc Interv 2003;60(2):221–3.

A Cardiologist's Perspective on Patent Foramen Ovale-Associated Conditions

Bernhard Meier, MD, FACC, FESC*

KEYWORDS

- Patent foramen ovale • Stroke • Transient ischemic attack • Myocardial infarction • Migraine
- Device closure • Mechanical vaccination • Primary prevention

KEY POINTS

- Patent foramen ovale is dramatically underdiagnosed as a cause of medical problems, including death.
- Patent foramen ovale is the cardiac problem that is easiest to solve, because closing a patent foramen ovale is the simplest and safest intervention in cardiology.
- Percutaneous closure of the foramen ovale is cardiology's catheter-based intervention with the best clinical yield.
- Closure of a patent foramen ovale represents a mechanical vaccination against a number of major and minor problems.
- Closure of the foramen ovale is mainly, albeit not exclusively, a preventive procedure.

 Video content accompanies this article at http://www.cardiology.theclinics.com.

INTRODUCTION

The first case reported incriminating the patent foramen ovale (PFO) as a cause of a clinical event dates back to the nineteenth century and ended fatally.[1] Based on the fact that the prevalence of PFO carriers decreases with age, it was later claimed that the PFO can close spontaneously anytime during lifetime.[2] That is hard to believe. A selective mortality of PFO carriers is a more likely explanation.[3]

The PFO still does not get the medical attention it deserves. In the early 90s, pediatric cardiologists started to percutaneously close PFOs with devices developed for closure of mid-size atrial septal defects.[4] On September 10, 1997, I implanted the world's first dedicated PFO device.[5] It was the Amplatzer PFO Occluder, developed by Kurt Amplatz, MD. This technique proved to be simple, safe, and efficacious from the very beginning. It is 1 of just 2 techniques in interventional cardiology that have never needed and therefore have never seen significant device modifications since their first clinical use. The other device is the Inoue balloon for mitral valvuloplasty.[6] Considering that PFO closure eliminates potentially life-threatening problems and has an almost 100% technical success rate, a close-to-zero complication rate, and a long-term clinical success rate of about 95%, it is difficult to understand that it is not used more frequently. Add to this that it is an outpatient procedure which takes normally about 15 minutes and that the patient needs no sedation during the intervention, feels no pain, can walk out of the catheterization laboratory holding the puncture site with a finger just like after donating blood,

University of Bern, Bern, Switzerland
* Nussbaumweg 40, Spiegel bei Bern 3095, Switzerland.
E-mail address: bernhard.meier@gmx.net

Cardiol Clin 42 (2024) 547–557
https://doi.org/10.1016/j.ccl.2024.02.002
0733-8651/24/© 2024 Elsevier Inc. All rights reserved.

can engage in all physical activities including sports as early as a few hours after the procedure, keeps the mark of a skin nick in the groin as only scar, and needs to take but some antiplatelet treatment for a couple of months. This sounds more like fixing a tooth than like a cardiac intervention. In light of its main purpose to protect the patient from later events, such as cerebral, coronary, ophthalmic, visceral, or peripheral paradoxic embolism, and because of the fact that it does this reliably and for life, the fitting term "mechanical vaccination" has been coined.[7]

SCOPE OF THE PROBLEM

For unknown reasons and irrationally, the PFOs potential to do harm remains considered by many as limited to cerebral embolic events in otherwise healthy people. Such events were and still are erroneously called cryptogenic, irrespective of whether a PFO was screened for or found.[8] Strokes in the realm of atrial fibrillation (AF) were in the beginning also subsumed under the then new term cryptogenic. Eventually, AF but not the PFO was upgraded to an established stroke cause joining atherosclerosis of cerebral vessels. It is blatantly ignored that a PFO with aggravating characteristics has a higher risk for causing a stroke than paroxysmal AF with rare and short episodes (**Fig. 1**). Plus, both PFO and AF typically are but presumptive culprits of embolic stroke. The actual source of cerebral emboli is, with few exceptions,[9,10] virtually never traceable. **Box 1** proposes a stroke classification paying respect to these facts and urging to give up the term cryptogenic in favor of the term embolic stroke of undetermined source (ESUS)[8] and placing it at the very tail of the list.

   As a consequence of the bizarre but prevalent classification of PFO as a cause exclusively for cryptogenic strokes, all the comparative and randomized studies, and hence the available data, on PFO and stroke dealt so far with young and otherwise healthy patients. The PFO cannot selectively let clots pass exclusively in people who are young and have no other stroke causes, can it? On the contrary, the sicker and older people get, the more likely are they to harbor thrombi in their veins.[11] Venous thrombi are the prerequisite of paradoxic embolism through a PFO. Add to this that a Valsalva maneuver, the classical PFO spreader, is more common in sick and old people due to defecation and micturition problems, chronic coughs, and so forth. Closing a PFO is so simple and innocuous (**Fig. 2**) that age and comorbidity have little, if any, influence on its ease, risk, or success. Hence, the older and sicker a

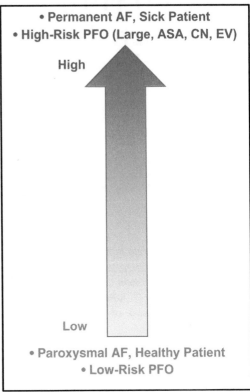

Fig. 1. Stroke risk according to the type of atrial fibrillation (AF) or patent foramen ovale (PFO). ASA, atrial septal aneurysm; CN, Chiari network; EV, Eustachian valve.

patient with a PFO is, the higher the absolute clinical yield of closure and the more pressing to close it.[12] The current guidelines shamefully claim the opposite.

   PFO closure is currently an accepted indication solely for people under the age of 65 (for some even 60) years with a history of an ischemic event (that for many has to be cerebral) and no other findable cause for it. There are plenty of randomized data for this indication but none for any other preventive indication or for the elderly. It sounds more than reasonable to extrapolate the randomized data and assume that ischemic events can also be prevented in the elderly by this mechanical vaccination. In fact, the absolute number of prevented events per patient and time will be higher in light of the more common preventable events. At all ages, it is cynical for people at risk to be told that they have to wait for their event before this simple and effective preventive procedure will be done, because there are no data on primary prevention. The first event may be a debilitating stroke or even death. Not long ago, in some

Box 1
Stroke classification

- Arterial occlusion
  - Lacunar
  - Intracerebral
  - Vertebral
  - Internal carotid
  - Common carotid
  - Brachiocephalic
- *Cryptogenic* (initial ranking)
  - Arterial embolus from
    - Plaque/ulcer/dissection
      - Intracerebral
      - Carotid
      - Vertebral
      - Brachiocephalic
      - Ascending aortic
  - Cardiac embolus from
    - Left ventricle
    - Left atrium
      - Left atrial appendage (atrial fibrillation)
      - Left atrial foramen pouch
    - Myxoma or other tumor
    - Vegetation (septic embolus)
- *Cryptogenic* (more recent ranking)
  - Paradoxic embolus via/from
    - Patent foramen ovale
    - Atrial septal defect
    - Pulmonary fistula
  - *Pulmonary venous bed embolus*
- *Cryptogenic* (correct ranking, better use: ESUS)

overall yield regarding positive minus negative effects? Think of the countless events in control groups of further randomized trials that could and should be prevented rather than just watched and counted in a trial.[15] Equally importantly, the positive effects for a given indication always include as collateral benefits the positive effects of all other indications. Close a PFO for migraine and the patient is vaccinated for life against paradoxic embolism into the cerebral or coronary arteries. Inversely, close a PFO after a cerebral event and the patient may be cured from migraine. How about that?

Patent Foramen Ovale Closure for Secondary Prevention

Stroke and transient ischemic attack

Regarding indications for PFO closure, one should not make a difference between stroke and TIA (see **Box 2**). A TIA is just a stroke in a patient with luck. The argument that a TIA may be a misinterpreted migraine attack falls short of the mark. PFO closure is a good therapy for migraine while at the same time protecting against future real strokes. Even less should one acquit the PFO based on the mere fact that there are other potential stroke causes present or the patient is old. The absolute risk that the PFO was the actual culprit is higher in such patients than in the young and so-called cryptogenic stroke patients. Only the relative risk is lower. AF is commonly considered a contraindication to PFO closure. That is wrong in 3 ways. First, even if patients with AF are under chronic oral anticoagulation (OAC), PFO closure should be performed. Paradoxic embolism is more common in patients with AF than in completely healthy people, for the very reason that they are not completely healthy people. PFO closure puts an end to paradoxic embolism once and for all; OAC does not. It just reduces the risk. Second, a complex search for occult AF in young and otherwise healthy patients with a stroke makes no sense. The yield is minute and even if AF is found, it was hardly the culprit for the stroke and certainly not the prime suspect in the presence of a high-risk PFO (see **Fig. 1**). Most importantly, it irresponsibly defers PFO closure and often defers it indefinitely or at least until the next event. The patient and the doctors in charge simply forget that the initial plan was to search for AF for 6 months or a year and then close the PFO if no AF is found. Third, the most elegant and best approach is to close the PFO and the left atrial appendage (LAA), laying to rest OAC and improving the life

countries, people who had had a first event had to wait for a second event while taking blood thinners to qualify for PFO closure. This was outright macabre.

Box 2 lists the current indications for PFO closure, all with some supportive data.[3] Statistically significant positive randomized data are available exclusively for ischemic events[13] and migraine.[14] Yet, should we not extrapolate randomized data without actually collecting them for cardiology's simplest procedure with the best

Intricacy of Intervention

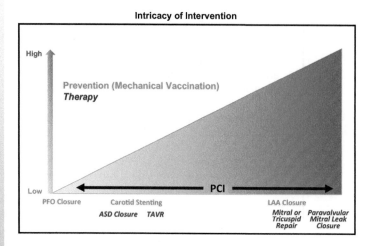

Fig. 2. Intricacy of interventional procedures in adult cardiology. ASD, atrial septal defect; LAA, left atrial appendage; PFO, patent foramen ovale; TAVR, transcatheter aortic valve replacement.

expectancy 2-fold. PFO closure[16] and LAA closure[17,18] have shown to prolong life.

Myocardial infarction

MI by paradoxic embolism through a PFO is a dramatically underdiagnosed problem.[19] It is perfectly preventable by PFO closure. For this largely ignored indication for PFO closure, the cardiologists are to blame. Like the neurologists illogically look for all other potential causes for stroke before investigating the PFO, the cardiologists look for all other potential causes for an MI, such as spontaneous coronary dissection, protracted spasm, vasospastic compounds, or any kind of atherosclerosis before contemplating paradoxic embolism, which almost always comes through a PFO. Again, the more atherosclerosis and the older and sicker the patient, the more likely becomes paradoxic embolism of a venous clot, and not the other way around. Many an interventional cardiologist has never pondered a PFO as the cause for MI. Making the mathematics, the amount of blood per minute reaching the coronary arteries corresponds to almost a third of that reaching the brain. Both territories are vulnerable to small clots passing through a PFO in contrast to visceral organs or limbs where only larger clots are relevant. After correcting for silent brain areas and collateralized coronary areas, we should diagnose roughly 1 PFO-mediated MI per 3 PFO-mediated cerebral events. Come to think of it, even more because our neurology colleagues drastically underdiagnose PFO-mediated cerebral events as discussed earlier. We need to improve our respective diagnostic accuracy at least 100-fold. If there is an acute MI with a blockage that looks even remotely embolic, swiftly open the coronary artery with primary percutaneous coronary intervention and then immediately look for a PFO with a right heart

catheter and close it if found. This adds 15 minutes to your case (not really a problem even at night time) and it does not measurably increase the overall risk but does a lot of good, even if that particular MI was not caused by the PFO. The next one might be and remember the collateral benefit of the mechanical vaccination. Screening for a PFO with a right heart catheter in a patient who is being catheterized for another reason is as accurate and less uncomfortable for the patient than screening for a PFO with transesophageal echocardiography (TEE). To account for the remote possibility that part of a clot could still be trapped in the PFO in an acute setting,[9] a distant contrast medium injection from the entrance of the right atrium is advised to start the search for the PFO (**Fig. 3**). The characteristics of the PFO needed to select the appropriate device size can be equally well documented with such a contrast medium injection as with TEE. The patient is optimally served with a combined coronary intervention and PFO closure.

Patent Foramen Ovale Closure for Primary Prevention

High-risk patent foramen ovale

PFO closure for primary prevention deserves to be put on the agenda urgently (see **Box 2**). First, it should be offered for people who for whatever reason are known to have a high-risk PFO. Not to forget, the term high-risk encompasses in addition to PFOs with high-risk features, every PFO that is presumed to have already caused an ischemic event. In the realm of primary prevention, a high-risk PFO is a PFO with an unprovoked right-to-left shunt, a PFO associated with a flimsy septum primum, also called atrial septal aneurysm (ASA),[20] with a Eustachian valve,[21] or with a Chiari network. An ASA briefly opens the PFO practically

Box 2
Indications for patent foramen ovale closure

- Secondary prevention
  - Stroke
  - Transient ischemic attack
  - Embolic myocardial infarction
  - Takotsubo
  - Peripheral embolism
  - Decompression incident
  - Mountain sickness
- Primary prevention
  - Aggravating PFO attributes (high-risk PFO)
    - Atrial septal aneurysm
    - Eustachian valve
    - Chiari network
  - Hypercoagulability
  - Deep venous thrombosis
  - Pulmonary embolism
  - Pacemaker/defibrillator electrodes
  - Right heart catheters
  - Surgery
    - Any major
    - Orthopedic
    - Cerebral in sitting position
  - Planned pregnancy
  - Carcinoid tumor
  - Special congenital/genetic situations
- Therapeutic
  - Migraine (particularly with aura)
  - Vasospastic angina
  - Platypnea–orthodeoxia
  - Exercise desaturation
  - Sleep apnea
- Vocational or recreational
  - Deep sea diver
  - Mountain climber, highlander
  - Brass musician
  - Glass blower
  - Tile setter
  - Military jet or acrobat pilot
  - Astronaut

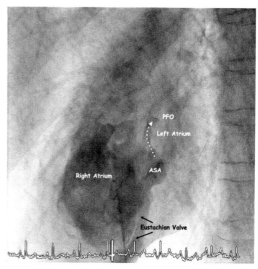

Fig. 3. Angiographic screening for and documentation of a patent foramen ovale (PFO) in a lateral projection. All important PFO characteristics are visible, such as the location and the width of the PFO (*dotted arrow*), the atrial septal aneurysm (ASA), and the Eustachian valve.

with every heart beat and creates considerable overall time that there is a right to left shunt. A Eustachian valve or a Chiari network escorts the clots from the inferior vena cava (where they all come from) directly through the PFO. All these features are associated with a high PFO prevalence because they hinder and often prevent PFO closure in the first year of life.

Family history, coagulation disorders, or thromboembolic disease
Other candidates for PFO closure for primary prevention are people with a close blood relative, for example, twin, having suffered a PFO-mediated stroke or MI and patients with hypercoagulability,[22] thrombophilia,[23] or a tendency to deep venous thrombosis and pulmonary embolism. This includes such patients who are under OAC. OAC protects only partially and rather poorly in the presence of the common compliance issues or during medically imposed pauses. PFO closure, by definition, knows no compliance issues or pauses.

Major surgery
Patients undergoing major surgical operations should be screened for a PFO and pretreated with closure if they have a PFO and there is time.[24] Closing the PFO reduces the risk of a stroke within the first year from 9% to 1%. Some neurosurgeons like to operate on sitting patients for reduced venous bleeding thanks to gravity.

That should not be done without having looked for a PFO before and closed it, if present.[25] Air can be sucked in through skull or brain veins opened during surgery. Via a PFO, air might bypass the lung filter and directly access the systemic circulation. Air is lighter than blood and will invariably return to the highest area in the sitting patient, that is, the brain.

Carcinoid tumor

Patients with a carcinoid tumor have a higher risk of left heart valve problems if they have a PFO.[26] This risk is reduced after PFO closure. Serotonin produced by the tumor is detrimental to heart valves in high doses. It gets neutralized before reaching the left heart valves if it has to pass through the lung filter, but not if it can bypass the lung through a PFO.

Therapeutic Patent Foramen Ovale Closure

Migraine

Migraine represents the most common and compelling situation where therapeutic rather than simply preventive PFO closure is considered (see **Box 2**). Theory has it that a metabolic trigger like serotonin, with its typical high concentration in venous blood and low concentration in arterial blood after neutralization in the lung filter, may pass through the PFO in a gush. An ensuing serotonin tsunami in the systemic circulation may then activate a single or a couple of hypersensitive receptors in the brain vessels causing a cortical spreading depression.[27] This results in a headache commonly preceded by an aura. If only a single hypersensitive receptor exists or all hypersensitive receptors are located in the same hemisphere, the migraine symptoms regularly occur in an identical manner or at least on the same side.

The approach to PFO closure in migraine patients provides another classic example of how evidence-based medicine can be misinterpreted to the disadvantage of patients.[15] There is uniform agreement about the increased prevalence of PFOs among migraine patients[28] and the increased prevalence of migraine among people with a PFO.[29] The still prevailing opinion that this just means that some common genes cause both migraine and the persistence of a PFO becomes untenable because PFO closure improves some migraines. Indeed, all comparative trials, nonrandomized or randomized, showed a numerical benefit of PFO closure compared to medical treatment alone in patients with migraine, particularly but not exclusively in those with aura.[30] In most nonrandomized comparisons, the significance was statistically significant. Unfortunately, the arbitrarily chosen primary endpoints of all 3 major randomized trials, while showing numerical benefits, failed the predefined statistical significance threshold. The complexity of the migraine patients included (all were required to have had several previous failed therapy approaches), overly ambitious primary endpoints, and the blunting placebo effect in the studies with sham procedures accounted for that. Of note, most of the secondary endpoints showed statistically significant superiority of PFO closure. Focusing on the failed primary endpoints and the fact that the trials were designed for superiority, the neurologic societies unanimously and mistakenly declared PFO closure as no valid alternative to medical treatment for migraine. They claimed that evidence-based medicine requires statistically significant benefits to change from an established to a new therapy. That is not entirely true because evidence-based medicine leaves room for interpretation. Common sense should conclude from the data that adopting PFO closure as a new therapy for migraine is certain to not disadvantage patients. Quite to the contrary, it will offer them a fair chance of benefitting. Add to this that a single intervention, that is, a mechanical vaccination, as simple and safe as PFO closure, should be preferred to long-term drugs with ever accumulating side effects and accruing cost for decades, if not for life.

An embargo on PFO closure in patients with migraine still prevails in neurology circles, and it can also be found among general practitioners caring for migraine patients and even among cardiologists. This questionable attitude direly neglects the mentioned fact that PFO closure in patients with migraine protects, as a collateral benefit, patients lifelong against paradoxic embolism, leading to stroke, MI, or even death. It also ignores meta-analyses of the published randomized trials,[31] most importantly the one done on an individual patient basis.[14] They unequivocally prove statistically significant advantages of PFO closure in migraine in virtually all relevant endpoints.

A modern and affordable approach to migraine and PFO is to screen patients with typical migraine for a PFO, then close the PFO if found and enjoy together with at least half the patients the immediate and sustained migraine improvement as well as together with all the patients the once and for all protection against paradoxic embolism.

The horrible destiny of a 39 year old nurse rests deeply engraved into my memory. I saw her 2 years after she had suffered a stroke that left her aphasic. She had to carry on to educate her 2 teenage sons and to function in her social and professional environments, and she continued to have frequent debilitating migraine attacks like she had known them for decades before her stroke. I closed her PFO and the migraine disappeared. The aphasia persisted, of course. Had I known her before her stroke and closed her PFO for migraine, she would not only have got rid of the crippling migraine earlier but she would not have her stroke. She would still be talking.

Vasospastic angina
Vasospastic angina mediated by a PFO can be explained by serotonin tsunamis, just like migraine. PFO closure improves that.[27]

Platypnea–orthodeoxia
Especially in elderly and obese patients, a sitting position pushes the diaphragm cranially. It is assumed that this may deform the heart in a way that the PFO opens widely. This leads to significant arterial desaturation that is immediately reversible by assuming a supine position and is called platypnea–orthodeoxia syndrome.[32,33] The syndrome is accompanied by an increased risk of paradoxic embolism of thrombotic material. PFO closure solves both problems.

Exercise desaturation
A similar situation called exercise desaturation occurs in some people during strenuous physical activities. The PFO opens persistently, causes cyanosis, and limits the exercise capacity substantially.[33] The phenomenon appears to be quite common in people with PFO. A report on 50 people with a PFO found exercise desaturation in a third. The problem was improved by PFO closure.[34]

Sleep apnea
Sleep apnea can be obstructive or central.[35] The obstructive type leads to increased venous backflow into the thorax during prolonged inspiration phases. This opens a PFO if present and not only increases the risk of paradoxic embolism but also aggravates central sleep apnea by the desaturation ensuing from the PFO being in a prolonged open position.[36–38] PFO closure improves that.

Patent Foramen Ovale Closure for Vocational or Recreational Reasons

Deep sea diving
Diving carries a risk for decompression accidents (see **Box 2**). A PFO increases that risk significantly.[39] Divers suffer more cerebral events and have more lacunar brain lesions on MRI if they have a PFO.[40] PFO closure is effective in preventing recurrent decompression events.[39]

Mountain climbing and living at high altitude
Mountain climbing harbors the risk of high-altitude cerebral and pulmonary edema, also known as acute mountain sickness. A PFO increases that risk[41,42] and PFO closure merits a chance to prove that it can remedy that problem. Highlanders develop elevated right atrial pressures. They react to low oxygen concentrations of the ambient air with chronic constriction of pulmonary arterioles to the end of prolonging blood passage through the lungs in order to optimize oxygen transfer to the erythrocytes. Elevated right atrial pressure corresponds to the situation at the release of a Valsalva maneuver and opens the PFO. Highlanders with a PFO are at increased risk for paradoxic embolism and a permanent right-to-left shunt through a PFO worsens the situation. It decreases oxygen saturation in the blood and leads to more constriction of the pulmonary arterioles and even higher right atrial pressure. A vicious cycle, if there ever was one.

Activities prone to Valsalva situations
Brass musicians and glass blowers are the salient examples of people using Valsalva maneuvers for work. People working in crouching positions or being exposed to high accelerations can also be counted in this group. Those individuals with a PFO are more prone to oxygen desaturation and paradoxic embolism during their work.

Screening for Patent Foramen Ovale

Screening for a PFO with closure for primary prevention in mind can wait for late adolescence. Before, there is practically no risk for venous thrombosis, without which the PFO is harmless. PFO-mediated embolic events in children are an exquisite rarity. Girls on contraceptives are the youngest group of people in whom the PFO may become a threat. Young people with migraine present an indication for PFO screening. Here, PFO closure as possible therapy should be considered, enhanced by primary prevention against later paradoxic embolism as a collateral bonus.

How can you screen for candidates who would benefit most from PFO closure in primary prevention? An interesting approach has been published in 2013,[43] but it has not been further pursued. An oximeter clamp was attached to the ear lobe and the person, divers in the study, performed a sustained Valsalva maneuver. Upon release of the Valsalva maneuver, a high-risk PFO will open briefly and a wave of venous blood will rush through the systemic circulation, passing the ear lobe. The oxygen saturation showed a dip in divers with a PFO but not in the others. The magnitude of the dip corresponded to the TEE-assessed PFO size.

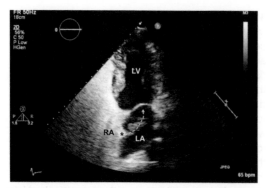

Fig. 4. Screening for a patent foramen ovale (PFO) with contrast transthoracic echocardiography. The high-risk PFO is evident by the large shunt (*dotted arrow*) and the atrial septal aneurysm (*asterisk*). LA, left atrium; LV, left ventricle; RA, right atrium.

Screening with such a test could be carried out in school classes or shopping malls. There, contrast echocardiography or transcranial Doppler (TCD) tests cannot be performed. They require a venous access. Even less can contrast TEE.

Short of such a simple, practical, and commercialized test with reproducible and validated results, transthoracic contrast echocardiography is our best option. It requires an echocardiography machine, a venous line, and an experienced 2-person team. It can be performed in most cardiology offices and in all hospitals with a cardiology service. It will miss small PFOs in contrast to TEE and TCD, but it will find all high-risk PFOs with the rare exception of the patients with no suitable echocardiographic window. **Fig. 4** and Video 1 show an example. TCD is an alternative, but it does not distinguish between PFO-mediated and pulmonary right-to-left shunts.

DISCUSSION

It is about time that closure of the PFO steps out of its Cinderella role and assumes a place in the limelight at the front of the stage. For about $ 50,000 in the United States and $ 10,000 or less in many other countries, an intervention, regarding complexity somewhere between implanting a loop recorder and implanting a pacemaker, can permanently solve several potential and actual problems in the role of a mechanical vaccination. I know of no other cardiac intervention that within less than an hour can prevent strokes, MIs, and death while at the same time improve symptoms like headaches and exertional or positional shortness of breath. On top of that, the psychological gain can be tremendous in some people.

There are insufficient medical capacity and funding to screen and treat 5% of the population with a high-risk PFO, not to mention the 25% of all PFO carriers. However, every situation bringing the PFO to mind should be grasped for a workup in this respect. Neurologists must recognize the fact that a PFO may be the culprit of any cerebral event or migraine. Cardiologists should look for a PFO and close it with every MI that was possibly caused by coronary embolism. Reimbursement should be ascertained for people who are sensitized to the PFO issue and want to know about their own situation, expecting that if they have a PFO it will be taken care of.

Major and minor myths about the PFO that need to be buried.

1. *The PFO risk is limited to the young and healthy.*
   The old and sick even have higher absolute risk.
2. *It is safe to wait for the first event before PFO closure.*
   The first event may have irreversible sequelae or even be fatal.
3. *AF is an important side effect of PFO closure.*
   AF virtually never occurs in a way requiring sustained treatment, except for patients already at the brink of AF before PFO closure.
4. *OAC and antiplatelets protect equally well as PFO closure.*
   That is only true for chronic OAC which is less elegant than a mechanical vaccination and

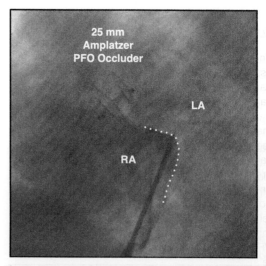

Fig. 5. Transseptal puncture after device closure of a patent foramen ovale. There is a large area safe for a transseptal puncture (*dotted line*) in the septum primum part of the fossa ovalis caudal to the fluoroscopically visible PFO device (left anterior oblique projection showing the device in perfect profile with no disc overlap). LA, left atrium; PFO, patent foramen ovale; RA, right atrium.

keeps on accumulation bleeding complications.

5. *PFO closure is heart surgery.*

   PFO closure is a very simple and innocuous outpatient procedure with no suffering or scar and negligible inconveniences before and after.

6. *PFO closure needs intraprocedural guiding by ultrasound imaging.*

   At least for the Amplatzer device, PFO closure under fluoroscopy is so simple, innocuous, and successful that ultrasound guidance cannot improve on that.

7. *PFO closure will prohibit later left atrial access for catheter-based interventions such as ablation for AF, LAA closure, or mitral valve interventions.*

   If anything, prior PFO closure facilitates a transseptal puncture under solely angiographic guidance (**Fig. 5**).[44]

8. *TCD is the only Doppler-based screening technique for PFO next to echocardiography with a bubble test.*

   TCD is a good but unnecessarily complicated and expensive technique for PFO screening. Rather than using a high-end ultrasound apparatus to target intracranial arteries, every extracranial artery or a finger artery accessible with a cheap ultrasound probe will do. Any bubble reaching a finger can also reach the brain and vice versa.

SUMMARY

The PFO represents a hitherto negligently underestimated and insufficiently worked up and treated cardiovascular health hazard. It is the simplest, safest, and cheapest to eliminate risk factor and medical problem in cardiology. PFO closure is mainly a preventive intervention, comparable to a mechanical vaccination. This vaccination is at the same time therapeutically effective in a significant proportion of patients with PFO-related symptoms or PFO-related events. The collateral benefit goes both ways. Close a PFO to prevent a given PFO-related problem and profit from improved symptoms of other PFO-related problems. Close a PFO to improve symptoms of a given PFO-related problem and get prevention against all other PFO-related problems. A PFO is present in roughly 25% of people, its particularly dangerous forms in about 5%. At least for the latter group, screening for and closure of the PFO as primary prevention will prevent events and be cost-effective. As a first step, it must get generally accepted and reflected in guidelines that the

PFO is a serious culprit candidate in any cerebral and coronary event that could be embolic, irrespective of age or accompanying disease. In contrast to common belief, the sicker and older the patient is, the higher is the absolute probability that the PFO be the cause. It is unlikely to ever have to regret having closed a PFO, but it is likely to regret not having closed a PFO.

CLINICS CARE POINTS

- The patent foramen ovale (PFO) is proved to be causative in systemic embolic events.
- The absolute risk of a PFO increases with age and concomitant disease; only the relative risk decreases.
- The PFO can cause chronic reversible symptoms such as migraine, exertional dyspnea, and platypnea–orthodeoxia.
- PFO-related problems are grossly underdiagnosed in neurology and cardiology.
- The PFO is the simplest and safest procedure of interventional cardiology with the best overall yield.
- The potential benefit of PFO closure is underexploited in secondary prevention and still ignored in primary prevention.
- It is unlikely to ever have to regret having closed a PFO, but it is likely to regret not having closed a PFO.

DISCLOSURE

No conflicts of interest.
No funding received.

SUPPLEMENTARY DATA

Supplementary data related to this article can be found online at https://doi.org/10.1016/j.ccl.2024.02.002.

REFERENCES

1. Cohnheim J. A handbook for practitioners and students. London: The New Sydenham Society; 1889.
2. Hagen PT, Scholz DG, Edwards WD. Incidence and size of patent foramen ovale during the first 10 decades of life: an autopsy study of 965 normal hearts. Mayo Clin Proc 1984;59:17–20.
3. Meier B, Nietlispach F. The evil of the patent foramen ovale: we are seeing but the tip of the iceberg. Eur Heart J 2018;39(18):1650–2.

4. Bridges ND, Hellenbrand W, Latson L, et al. Transcatheter closure of patent foramen ovale after presumed paradoxical embolism. Circulation 1992; 86(6):1902–8.

5. Madhkour R, Meier B. Patent foramen ovale closure, a contemporary review. Structural Heart 2018;2(2): 114–20.

6. Inoue K, Owaki T, Nakamura T, et al. Clinical application of transvenous mitral commissurotomy by a new balloon catheter. J Thorac Cardiovasc Surg 1984; 87(3):394–402.

7. Meier B. Closure of the patent foramen ovale with dedicated Amplatzer occluders: closing in on a mechanical vaccination. Catheter Cardiovasc Interv 2008;72(1):80–1.

8. Elgendy AYSJ, Amin Z, Boudoulas KD, et al. Proposal for updated nomenclature and classification of potential causative mechanism in patent foramen ovale-associated stroke. JAMA Neurol 2020;77(7): 878–86.

9. Koullias GJ, Elefteriades JA, Wu I, et al. Images in cardiovascular medicine. Massive paradoxical embolism: caught in the act. Circulation 2004;109: 3056–7.

10. Parekh A, Jaladi R, Sharma S, et al. Images in cardiovascular medicine. The case of a disappearing left atrial appendage thrombus: direct visualization of left atrial thrombus migration, captured by echocardiography, in a patient with atrial fibrillation, resulting in a stroke. Circulation 2006;114(13):e513–4.

11. Anderson FA Jr, Wheeler HB, Goldberg RJ, et al. A population-based perspective of the hospital incidence and case-fatality rates of deep vein thrombosis and pulmonary embolism. The Worcester DVT Study. Arch Intern Med 1991;151:933–8.

12. Mazzucco S, Li L, Rothwell PM. Prognosis of cryptogenic stroke with patent foramen ovale at older ages and implications for trials: a population-based study and systematic review. JAMA Neurol 2020;77(10): 1279–87.

13. Kent DMSJ, Kasner SE, Nelson J, et al. Heterogeneity of treatment effects in an analysis of pooled individual patient data from randomized trials of device closure of patent foramen ovale after stroke. JAMA 2021;326(22):2277–86.

14. Mojadidi MKKP, Mahmoud AN, Elgendy IY, et al. Pooled analysis of PFO occluder device trials in patients with PFO and migraine. J Am Coll Cardiol 2021;77(6):667–76.

15. Meier B, Nietlispach F. Fallacies of evidence-based medicine in cardiovascular medicine. Am J Cardiol 2019;123(4):690–4.

16. Wahl A, Jüni P, Mono ML, et al. Long-term propensity score-matched comparison of percutaneous closure of patent foramen ovale with medical treatment after paradoxical embolism. Circulation 2012; 125:803–12.

17. Reddy VY, Sievert H, Halperin J, et al. Percutaneous left atrial appendage closure vs warfarin for atrial fibrillation: a randomized clinical trial. JAMA 2014; 312:1988–98.

18. Gloekler S, Fürholz M, de Marchi S, et al. Left atrial appendage closure versus medical therapy in patients with atrial fibrillation: the APPLY study. EuroIntervention 2020;16(9):e767–74.

19. Raphael CE, Heit JA, Reeder GS, et al. Coronary embolus: an underappreciated cause of acute coronary syndromes. JACC Cardiovasc Interv 2018; 11(2):172–80.

20. Mas JL, Saver JL, Kasner SE, et al. Association of atrial septal aneurysm and shunt size with stroke recurrence and benefit from patent foramen ovale closure. JAMA Neurol 2022;79(11):1175–9.

21. Schuchlenz HW, Saurer G, Weihs W, et al. Persisting Eustachian valve in adults: relation to patent foramen ovale and cerebrovascular events. J Am Soc Echocardiogr 2004;17:231–3.

22. Buber J, Guetta V, Orion D, et al. Patent foramen ovale closure among patients with hypercoagulable states maintained on antithrombotic therapy. Cardiology 2021;146(3):375–83.

23. Liu K, Song B, Palacios IF, et al. Patent foramen ovale attributable cryptogenic embolism with thrombophilia has higher risk for recurrence and Responds to closure. JACC Cardiovasc Interv 2020; 13(23):2745–52.

24. Friedrich S, Ng PY, Platzbecker K, et al. Patent foramen ovale and long-term risk of ischaemic stroke after surgery. Eur Heart J 2019;40(11):914–24.

25. Fathi AR, Eshtehardi P, Meier B. Patent foramen ovale and neurosurgery in sitting position: a systematic review. Br J Anaesth 2009;102(5):588–96.

26. Douglas S, Oelofse T, Shah T, et al. Patent foramen ovale in carcinoid heart disease: the potential role for and risks of percutaneous closure prior to cardiothoracic surgery. J Neuroendocrinol 2023;35(8): e13323.

27. Ravi D, Tobis J, Parikh R, et al. A new syndrome of patent foramen ovale inducing vasospastic angina and migraine. J Am Coll Cardiol Case Reports 2024;28:102132.

28. Schwerzmann M, Nedeltchev K, Lagger F, et al. Prevalence and size of directly detected patent foramen ovale in migraine with aura. Neurology 2005;65: 1415–8.

29. Schwedt TJ, Demaerschalk BM, Dodick DW. Patent foramen ovale and migraine: a quantitative systematic review. Cephalalgia 2008;28(5):531–40.

30. Ben-Assa E, Rengifo-Moreno P, Al-Bawardy R, et al. Effect of residual interatrial shunt on migraine burden after transcatheter closure of patent foramen ovale. JACC Cardiovasc Interv 2020;13(3):293–302.

31. Kheiri B, Abdalla A, Osman M, et al. Percutaneous closure of patent foramen ovale in migraine: a

meta-analysis of randomized clinical trials. JACC Cardiovasc Interv 2018;11(8):816–8.

32. Hayek A, Rioufol G, Bochaton T, et al. Prognosis after percutaneous foramen ovale closure among patients with platypnea-orthodeoxia syndrome. J Am Coll Cardiol 2021;78(18):1844–6.

33. Mojadidi MK, Ruiz JC, Chertoff J, et al. Patent foramen ovale and hypoxemia. Cardiol Rev 2019; 27(1):34–40.

34. Devendra GP, Rane AA, Krasuski RA. Provoked exercise desaturation in patent foramen ovale & impact of percutaneous closure. J Am Coll Cardiol Intv 2012;5(4):416–9.

35. Oldenburg O. Cheyne-Stokes respiration in chronic heart failure, treatment with adaptive servoventilation therapy. Circ J 2012;76:2305–17.

36. Agnoletti G, Iserin L, Lafont A, et al. Obstructive sleep apnea and patent foramen ovale: successful treatment of symptoms by percutaneous foramen ovale closure. J Interv Cardiol 2005;18:393–5.

37. White JM, Veale AG, Ruygrok PN. Patent foramen ovale closure in the treatment of obstructive sleep apnea. J Invasive Cardiol 2013;25(8):E169–71.

38. Rimoldi SF, Ott S, Rexhaj E, et al. Patent foramen ovale closure in obstructive sleep apnea improves blood pressure and cardiovascular function. Hypertension 2015;66(5):1050–7.

39. Honek J, Sramek M, Honek T, et al. Patent foramen ovale closure is effective in divers: long-term results from the DIVE-PFO Registry. J Am Coll Cardiol 2020; 76(9):1149–50.

40. Billinger M, Zbinden R, Mordasini R, et al. Patent foramen ovale closure in recreational divers: effect on decompression illness and ischaemic brain lesions during long-term follow-up. Heart 2011;97:1932–7.

41. West BH, Fleming RG, Al Hemyari B, et al. Relation of patent foramen ovale to acute mountain sickness. Am J Cardiol 2019;123(12):2022–5.

42. Allemann Y, Hutter D, Lipp E, et al. Patent foramen ovale and high-altitude pulmonary edema. JAMA 2006;296(24):2954–8.

43. Billinger M, Schwerzmann M, Rutishauser W, et al. Patent foramen ovale screening by ear oximetry in divers. Am J Cardiol 2013;111:286–90.

44. Zaker-Shahrak R, Fuhrer J, Meier B. Transseptal puncture for catheter ablation of atrial fibrillation after device closure of patent foramen ovale. Catheter Cardiovasc Interv 2008;71:551–2.

Patent Foramen Ovale and Coronary Artery Spasm
A New Patent Foramen Ovale-associated Condition that May Explain the Mechanism of Vasospastic Angina

Deepak Ravi, MD[a], Rushi V. Parikh, MD[a], Jamil A. Aboulhosn, MD[b], Jonathan M. Tobis, MD[a],*

KEYWORDS

- Patent foramen ovale • Vasospastic angina • Angina with nonobstructive coronary arteries (ANOCA)
- Microvascular dysfunction • Migraine with aura • Takotsubo cardiomyopathy • Migraine
- Vasoactive substances

KEY POINTS

- Patent foramen ovale (PFO) may play a key role in the pathogenesis of migraine, vasospastic angina, and Takotsubo cardiomyopathy by permitting vasoactive substances to bypass the pulmonary circulation and pass into the systemic circulation.
- PFO closure may represent an effective therapeutic option in patients with the syndrome of PFO and vasospastic angina. Moreover, given the possible link between PFO and Takotsubo cardiomyopathy, PFO closure may help prevent the development of Takotsubo cardiomyopathy in susceptible patients with evidence of PFO and prior history of Takotsubo cardiomyopathy.
- Angina with nonobstructive coronary arteries (ANOCA) is a clinical spectrum that results in varying degrees of anginal chest pain despite the lack of obstructive coronary artery disease. ANOCA contributes significantly to health care utilization and results in increased morbidity and mortality to patients. Underlying mechanisms include functional endothelial dysregulation and/or coronary microvascular dysfunction.
- Invasive coronary function testing can help establish a diagnosis for patients with suspected ANOCA. Moreover, categorizing patients into phenotypic subgroups may further guide medical management of patients with ANOCA.

INTRODUCTION

Patent foramen ovale (PFO) has been associated with migraine, and particularly migraine with aura. PFO is thought to set the stage for migraines by permitting vasoactive substances to pass to the brain that are unfiltered by the pulmonary circulation. Several neuropeptides, including calcitonin gene-related peptide (CGRP), pituitary adenylate cyclase-activating polypeptide, and serotonin, have been implicated in the pathophysiology of migraine and are under investigation as potential therapeutic targets. For example, CGRP concentrations have been shown to be elevated in patients with chronic migraine and return to normal levels with triptan therapy.[1] Serotonin, which is a

[a] Department of Medicine, Division of Cardiology, University of California Los Angeles; [b] Department of Medicine, Division of Cardiology, University of California Los Angeles, Ahmanson/UCLA Adult Congenital Heart Center
* Corresponding author. 10833 LeConte Avenue, Los Angeles, CA 90095-1717.
E-mail address: Jtobis@mednet.ucla.edu

Cardiol Clin 42 (2024) 559–571
https://doi.org/10.1016/j.ccl.2024.02.003

prothrombotic, vasoactive substance that is usually metabolized in the pulmonary vasculature by monoamine oxidase, may further contribute to migraine development.[2] Studies have demonstrated reduction in serotonin levels after PFO closure.[3] Moreover, embolization of small platelet aggregates into the systemic circulation has been shown to induce focal transient ischemia of the cerebral circulation, which has been associated with migraine onset.[2] Whereas these prothrombotic and vasoactive substances would otherwise be cleared by the pulmonary circulation, in the presence of a PFO, they may enter the arterial system, inducing cortical spreading depression, and resulting in a migraine attack.[4,5] Several studies have supported this link between PFO and migraine, particularly in those with migraine with aura.[2] A systematic review of 12 case reports of PFO and migraine found an incidence of 46% to 88.0% in those with aura.[6] Furthermore, those with PFO have been found to be more likely to develop migraine with aura, with an odds ratio of developing migraine of 5.13.[2,7] Finally, those with larger PFOs appear to be at greater risk of developing migraine with aura, with the degree of shunting characterized by both transthoracic echocardiogram (TTE) with bubble study and transcranial Doppler (TCD).[2,8,9]

The use of antiplatelet agents, such as the P2Y12 inhibitors, may be effective in patients with drug-refractory migraine and PFO. In a study of 26 patients with migraine and PFO, the addition of clopidogrel to baseline medical therapy significantly reduced headache frequency and attack duration, with fewer visual auras and less migraine-associated disability.[10] A meta-analysis of 262 patients with migraine and 539 patients who were initiated on antiplatelet therapy for primary prevention of migraine after atrial septal defect (ASD) closure similarly demonstrated efficacy in reducing migraine symptoms with clopidogrel. In particular, patients with migraine who were treated with P2Y12 inhibitors had a pooled response rate of 0.64 (95% confidence interval [CI]: 0.43–0.81, $P = .005$). P2Y12 inhibitors also reduced the frequency of new-onset migraine in those undergoing ASD closure (odds ratio = 0.41, 95% CI: 0.22–0.77).[11] P2Y12 inhibitor use has also been studied in migraine after ASD closure. The CANOA trial evaluated the use of clopidogrel in addition to aspirin for the prevention of migraine attacks following ASD closure. Patients were randomized to receive dual antiplatelet therapy with aspirin and clopidogrel compared to aspirin alone (with a placebo). Patients in the clopidogrel group had a reduced number of migraine days and a lower incidence of migraine attacks following ASD closure.[12] These findings suggest platelet activation plays an important role in the pathogenesis of migraine.

Several studies have evaluated percutaneous PFO closure in the management of migraine with aura. The MIST trial (2008) evaluated patients with refractory migraine with 5 to 23 migraine days per month and utilized the STARFlex device. The primary endpoint used was the complete resolution of migraine, with the secondary endpoint of 50% reduction of headache days. There was no difference in the primary or secondary endpoints; however, there was a high frequency of residual shunting after closure, and the study population had a relatively low burden of symptoms (<5 days with migraine per month).[13] The PRIMA trial (2014) included patients with migraine with aura with greater than 3 migraine attacks or 5 migraine days per month, but fewer than 14 headache days per month. Further, all patients enrolled had documented evidence of PFO. The primary endpoint was the reduction in migraine days from baseline to 1 year after percutaneous closure with the Amplatzer device. The study was terminated early due to slow enrollment; however, there was a trend toward fewer migraine days, with a mean reduction in migraine days of 2.9 days in the closure group compared to 1.7 days in the medical therapy group.[14]

The PREMIUM trial (2017) was a double blind, sham-controlled trial that enrolled patients with 6 to 14 days of migraine per month, who were refractory to 3 different preventative medications. All patients were established to have a right-to-left shunt. The primary endpoint, arbitrarily required by the Food and Drug Administration (FDA), was "the responder rate," which was defined as the frequency of subjects who had a reduction in migraine attacks by 50% after percutaneous closure of PFO with the Amplatzer device (Abbott Cardiovascular, Chicago, IL). Since that trial, the FDA now accepts the number of migraine days per month as the primary endpoint for medication or device trials in migraine. In the PREMIUM trial, while there was a significant decrease in mean number of migraine days per month and in the number of patients who had complete cessation of migraine attacks (both secondary endpoints), the study did not meet its primary endpoint of responder rate.[15] Had the FDA agreed to use the number of migraine days, the endpoint of the PREMIUM trial would have been met and there would be approval today for PFO closure for migraine.

To further evaluate the efficacy and safety of percutaneous PFO closure in patients with migraine, Mojadidi and colleagues performed a pooled analysis of the PRIMA and PREMIUM trials.[16] In this analysis, the authors evaluated patient-level data from the PRIMA and PREMIUM trials and included all primary and secondary endpoints from both trials. All the endpoints were given equal importance. The endpoints included (1) mean reduction in monthly migraine days; (2) mean reduction in monthly migraine attacks; (3) responder rate (defined in earlier discussion); and (4) complete migraine cessation (100% reduction in migraine attacks during the treatment phase compared with the baseline phase). The authors also performed a subgroup analysis for patients with migraine with aura compared to those with migraine without aura, as it is postulated that patients with frequent aura may benefit more from percutaneous PFO closure. Safety outcomes, including procedural complications, were also reported for all patients who underwent percutaneous closure.

The study included data from 337 randomized patients (176 who underwent closure). The baseline characteristics did not vary significantly between the 2 groups, and the average number of migraine days (8.3 ± 3.1 days vs 8.2 ± 2.8 days; $P = .80$) and migraine attacks (4.9 ± 1.4 days vs 4.8 ± 1.8 days; $P = .59$) were largely similar. However, the PRIMA cohort had a higher number of patients with migraine with aura and higher Migraine Disability Assessment scores. The PREMIUM cohort had higher rates of mood disorders, palpitations, steroid use, and prior head trauma. With respect to effective closure rates, 3% of PRIMA patients had significant residual right-to-left shunt at 12 months on transesophageal echocardiogram (TEE), and 15% of PREMIUM patients had significant residual right-to-left shunt at 12 months on TCD. There was no difference in the change in migraine days (average number of migraine days 10–12 months post-PFO closure minus average number of migraine days 2 months pre-PFO closure) between those with no residual shunt and significant residual shunt.

The study found a significant reduction in monthly migraine days at 12 months between the closure group and the control group (-3.1 days ± 4.5 days vs -1.9 ± 4.2 days, $P = .02$). There was also a greater reduction in the mean number of migraine attacks in the PFO closure group (-2 ± 2.0 vs -1.4 ± 1.9; $P = .01$) and a higher rate of complete migraine cessation compared with medical therapy (9% vs 0.7%, $P < .001$). The responder rate (defined in earlier discussion) did not reach statistical significance but was met in 38% of the closure group and in 29% of the control ($P = .13$).

With respect to the subgroup of patients with migraine with aura, PFO closure resulted in a significant reduction in migraine days compared to the control group (-3.2 ± 4.8 days vs -1.8 ± 4.4 days; $P = .03$). However, those without aura did not have a significant reduction in migraine days (-2.8 ± 3.4 days vs -2.2 ± 4.0 days; $P = .53$). Complete headache cessation occurred in 11% of those with migraine with aura undergoing PFO closure but only in 0.9% of the control group ($P = .002$) but did not reach statistical significance in those without aura (5% vs 0%, $P = .16$). Interestingly, there was a significant reduction in the mean number of migraine attacks in those with (-2.0 ± 2.0 vs -1.4 ± 1.9, $P = .09$) and without aura (-2.0 ± 1.8 vs -1.0 ± 2.0, $P = .03$). This suggests that some patients without aura still may benefit from PFO closure.

Moreover, those with frequent aura (aura occurring in >50% of migraine attacks) had a greater reduction in migraine days (-4.3 ± 5.3 days vs -1.4 ± 4.8 days, $P = .002$), but those with infrequent aura had no significant reduction in migraine days (-2.4 ± 3.8 days vs -2.3 ± 3.7 day; $P = .99$). Again, complete headache cessation was significantly reduced in those with frequent aura undergoing PFO closure (13% vs 1.5%; $P = .01$) but was also significantly reduced in those with infrequent aura undergoing PFO closure (6% vs 0%, $P = .01$).

PFO closure was well tolerated with a total of 9 procedure-related adverse events and 4 device-related adverse events. The most common procedure-related adverse events included access-site hematoma and transient hypotension, and the most common device-related adverse event was paroxysmal atrial fibrillation.

This pooled analysis demonstrated a statistically significant reduction in migraine days in patients undergoing percutaneous PFO closure with the Amplatzer PFO Occluder device (**Fig. 1**). Patients with migraine with aura had a greater reduction in migraine days and higher likelihood of reaching complete migraine cessation with PFO closure. While those without aura did not have a significant reduction in migraine days, they did have a reduction in mean number of migraines, which suggests that migraineurs without aura may still benefit from PFO closure. As the pathophysiology of migraine is complex and multifactorial, migraineurs with PFO with aura and those without may share similar underlying factors and would still benefit from PFO closure. Further randomized controlled trials to evaluate PFO closure in various subsets of patients with migraine may help identify these underlying characteristics and identify those who would benefit from percutaneous PFO closure.

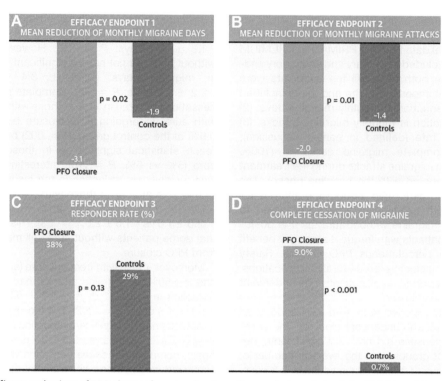

Fig. 1. Efficacy endpoints of PFO closure for migraine from the pooled analysis of the PRIMA and PREMIUM trials (reproduced with permission from Elsevier).

ANGINA WITH NONOBSTRUCTIVE CORONARY ARTERIES

Anginal chest pain is often ascribed to obstructive coronary artery disease; however, in up to 40% of patients, angiography does not reveal obstructive epicardial coronary artery disease.[17] Prinzmetal angina, first described by Prinzmetal as nonexertional angina that is not explained by a mismatch in myocardial oxygen consumption and mediated by vasospasm, is the most well-known manifestation of anginal chest pain in the absence of obstructive coronary artery disease. Further studies have elucidated other underlying processes that may contribute to the presence of angina with nonobstructive coronary artery disease. Collectively, this has been referred to as ANOCA, or in the presence of documented ischemia, ischemia with nonobstructive coronary arteries (INOCA). ANOCA/INOCA are understood to beget a spectrum of clinical syndromes, ranging from nonexertional and exertional chest pain to, in certain situations, even myocardial infarction (myocardial infarction with nonobstructive coronary arteries, MINOCA). Up to 5% to 10% of all myocardial infarctions may be attributed to MINOCA, and the 1-year all-cause mortality in MINOCA may be up to 3.5%.[18] ANOCA has been associated with significantly increased

cardiovascular risk, impaired quality of life, and increased health care utilization.

Several potential mechanisms may underlie the development of ANOCA. However, these processes primarily result in functional endothelial dysregulation resulting in coronary vasospasm (epicardial or microvascular) and/or coronary microvascular dysfunction (CMD).[5] Understanding the pathophysiologic basis of ANOCA can help tailor phenotype-specific therapies for various subsets of patients.

While the pathophysiology of functional endothelial dysregulation is poorly understood, a multifactorial process involving autonomic dysregulation, endothelial dysfunction, smooth muscle hyperreactivity, pre-existing atherosclerosis, and inflammation/oxidative stress has been hypothesized.[19] Endothelial nitric oxide appears to play a crucial role in preserving vascular tone. The loss of endothelial nitric oxide in the setting of oxidative stress may result in suboptimal vasodilation or even vasoconstriction in response to otherwise vasodilatory substances such as acetylcholine.[20] Furthermore, atherosclerosis and endothelial dysfunction are intrinsically linked, with atherosclerosis being shown to be closely linked with spasm in animal models.[20] This link has been demonstrated clinically as well, with one study demonstrating the presence of diffuse atherosclerosis or coronary calcification with intra-vascular ultrasound (IVUS) imaging in up to 80% of patients with ANOCA.[21]

CMD, on the other hand, refers to structural changes to the microcirculation in response to various stressors that ultimately increase the vascular tone. These changes include inward remodeling of coronary arterioles, resulting in increased wall to lumen ratio, and loss of myocardial capillary density. The increase in microvascular resistance results in decreased microcirculatory conductance and impaired oxygen delivery capacity, leading to anginal symptoms.[22] Risk factors associated with microvascular remodeling include smoking, hypertension, hyperlipidemia, diabetes, atherosclerosis, left ventricular hypertrophy, chronic inflammatory states, and primary and secondary cardiomyopathies.[19,20]

The diagnosis of ANOCA has historically been one of exclusion; however, developments in the measurement of coronary circulation have allowed for physiologic measurements that establish the diagnosis of coronary dysfunction. While the gold standard for physiologic measurement of coronary flow requires invasive measurements, several noninvasive methods may also provide information regarding coronary flow and the microvascular resistance. PET and cardiac MRI (cMRI) can measure surrogates for coronary flow. PET measures the change in radiotracer activity between the resting and hyperemic states and can infer coronary flow reserve (CFR). However, PET is not widely available due to its expense and the resources required. cMRI measures the T1 signal intensity that results from the diffusion of gadolinium from the microvasculature into the interstitial space, which is proportional to coronary perfusion and blood volume. This change in T1 signal intensity in turn can be used as a surrogate for CFR. The use of MRI-derived CFR needs further validation against invasive testing. Pulsed wave transthoracic Doppler echocardiography measures CFR at baseline and hyperemia but is only limited to assessing the left anterior descending artery, and its accuracy is highly operator dependent.[18]

Invasive coronary function testing (CFT) allows for direct measurement of the various components of the coronary vasculature. CFT typically involves the evaluation of the epicardial and microvasculature for evidence of vasospasm using acetylcholine provocation testing, as well as testing of the microvasculature for the presence of CMD using a pressure-thermistor coronary wire and coronary vasodilators.[19]

Acetylcholine is typically a potent vasodilator of the coronary vasculature. However, in the presence of endothelial dysfunction, due to an imbalance in the availability of nitric oxide, acetylcholine may result in epicardial or microvascular spasm. Epicardial coronary vasospasm is diagnosed when there is a reduction in lumen size (arbitrarily defined as 90% reduction in luminal diameter) with the administration of acetylcholine, with the reproduction of anginal chest pain. Typically, testing is performed with intracoronary administration of acetylcholine in the left anterior descending artery. Further evaluation of the epicardial arteries for the presence of myocardial bridging may be performed with intravascular ultrasound. Acetylcholine provocation testing is generally considered safe with a major complication rate of ~0.5%.[23]

PATENT FORAMEN OVALE AND VASOSPASTIC ANGINA

Coronary vasospasm is reversible constriction of the coronary vasculature. It is mediated by smooth muscle dysfunction, resulting in hypercontractility. Vasospastic angina occurs when there is enough narrowing of coronary arteries to compromise myocardial blood flow and cause symptoms. While the underlying mechanism mediating vasospastic angina has yet to be understood, hyperreactivity to vasoconstrictors and endothelial dysfunction are implicated.[24] PFO may play a key role in the development of angina in a subset of patients who are predisposed to smooth muscle hypercontractility. By permitting substances such as ergonovine, histamine, acetylcholine, and serotonin to pass into the coronary circulation, PFO may be a pathway that permits provocation of coronary vasospasm.[25] This proposed mechanism is depicted in further detail in **Fig. 2**.

A recently published case series described 9 women with PFO who also had migraine and vasospastic angina.[26] Seven of these patients had their PFO closed (6 with percutaneous closure, 1 with surgery), and all of them had resolution in their migraine and chest pain symptoms. Interestingly, 3 of the patients were sisters, suggesting a strong genetic predisposition as well. The first of the 3 sisters had a long-standing history of migraine with aura since childhood, and a 7 year history of intermittent chest pain. At the age of 49 years, the patient sought treatment of severe chest pain at an emergency department and then she developed ventricular fibrillation-cardiac arrest. After resuscitation, the patient underwent emergent cardiac catheterization, revealing focal narrowing of the LAD and a large diagonal vessel. The patient underwent balloon angioplasty because the physicians assumed that the coronary narrowing was due to atherosclerosis, but no stents were placed.

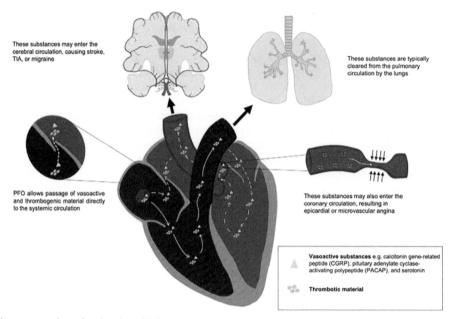

These substances may enter the cerebral circulation, causing stroke, TIA, or migraine

These substances are typically cleared from the pulmonary circulation by the lungs

PFO allows passage of vasoactive and thrombogenic material directly to the systemic circulation

These substances may also enter the coronary circulation, resulting in epicardial or microvascular angina

Vasoactive substances e.g. calcitonin gene-related peptide (CGRP), pituitary adenylate cyclase-activating polypeptide (PACAP), and serotonin

Thrombotic material

Fig. 2. The proposed mechanism by which PFO promotes coronary vasospasm, migraine, and transient ischemic attack (TIA)/stroke.

However, no intracoronary nitroglycerin was given to rule out vasospasm. Given her migraine history, she subsequently underwent TEE, which demonstrated a PFO. Repeat coronary angiography performed when the patient was chest pain free demonstrated normal coronary arteries with spontaneous reversal of the prior coronary narrowing, consistent with spasm. Intravascular ultrasound revealed no atherosclerosis or coronary calcification. Given resolution of the previously noted coronary artery narrowing, the patient was diagnosed with coronary vasospasm. Her PFO was closed percutaneously, and she has had no chest pain or migraines for 15 years since closure (**Fig. 3**).

The patient's 68-year-old sister developed chest pain after infection with coronavirus disease 2019 (COVID-19). She also had a long-standing history of migraine with aura. She underwent a thorough chest pain workup, including computed tomography (CT) pulmonary angiogram and coronary CT angiogram, which demonstrated no pulmonary embolism or coronary artery disease. However, a small PFO was noted. Given the largely unrevealing workup and her recent COVID-19 infection, the patient was presumed to have pericarditis and was treated with a course of nonsteroidal anti-inflammatory drugs. However, she developed recurrent chest discomfort and given her sister's history of chest pain associated with PFO, she underwent further workup for a shunt. A TCD demonstrated a Spencer grade 5/5 right-to-left shunt and

provocative testing for coronary vasospasm was pursued. Her baseline coronary angiogram was without any evidence of coronary artery disease; however, with administration of 100 μg of acetylcholine, the patient had significant vasospasm with angiographic evidence of luminal narrowing and had reproduction of her chest pain symptoms (**Fig. 4**). She subsequently underwent percutaneous PFO closure with a 25 mm Gore-Cardioform occluder device. She has had no recurrent chest pain or migraine since.

Similarly, 5 other patients aged 43 to 68 years with PFO, migraine, and vasospastic angina were described who underwent PFO closure with complete resolution of symptoms. Their presenting symptoms, workup, and clinical course are described in further detail in **Table 1**. Thus, the PFO pathway may represent a novel mechanism to explain the coronary vasospasm that occurs in ANOCA. If these observations are replicated in future studies of ANOCA, PFO closure may become a powerful intervention for those with PFO-associated coronary vasospasm. We do not know the frequency of PFO in patients with ANOCA, but this could be obtained easily in those centers that see many patients with ANOCA. Mechanistically, PFO closure eliminates the right-to-left shunting that may occur with an increased intrathoracic pressure. The elimination of the right-to-left shunt through the PFO forces all venous blood carrying vasoactive substances to pass through the pulmonary vasculature, where

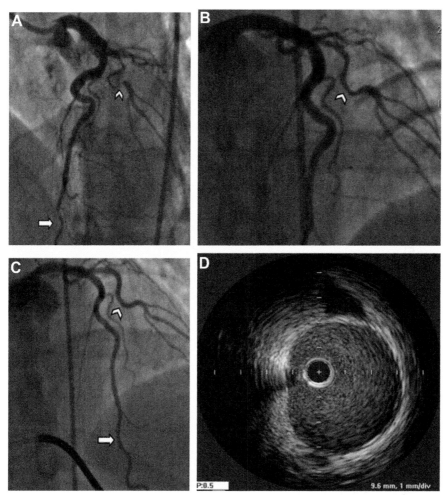

Fig. 3. (*A*) Angiogram demonstrated focal narrowing of the distal LAD (*arrow*) and more diffuse narrowing of the first diagonal artery (*caret*). (*B*) Angiogram after balloon angioplasty demonstrated persistent narrowing of the first diagonal artery. (*C*) Angiogram 6 months later demonstrated no evidence of coronary artery disease. (*D*) Intravascular ultrasound demonstrated no plaque in the LAD.

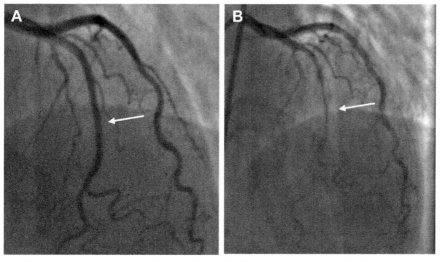

Fig. 4. (*A*) Baseline angiogram demonstrating angiographically normal LAD (*arrow*). (*B*) Angiogram after 100 μg acetylcholine I.C. demonstrating diffuse narrowing of the LAD (*arrow*).

Table 1
Clinical features of patients with clinical syndrome of migraine, vasospastic angina, and patent foramen ovale

	Case Presentation	Migraines	Chest Pain	PFO Evaluation	Angiography	Provocative Testing	PFO Closure	Medical Therapy	Residual Symptoms/ Length of Follow-up
1	49F with long-standing history of migraine with aura and intermittent angina for 7 y, who presented with chest pain and ventricular fibrillation	Yes	Yes	TEE	Index study with focal narrowing of distal LAD with repeat study demonstrating resolution of previously seen focal stenosis	No	Yes	Clopidogrel and ASA for 1 mo, ASA thereafter	No symptoms at 15 y follow-up; closed 2008
2	68F (sister of case 1) with several years of migraine with aura and recent onset angina after COVID-19 infection	Yes	Yes	TCD with 5/5 right-to-left shunt	No epicardial coronary artery disease	+Ach with narrowing of LAD (see **Fig. 1**)	Yes	Clopidogrel and ASA for 1 mo, ASA thereafter	No symptoms at 11 mo follow-up
3	38F with long-standing migraine history and 10 y of intermittent angina, found to have nocturnal hypoxemia to 80%	Yes	Yes	• TEE right-to-left shunting • TCD with 5/5 right-to-left shunt	No epicardial coronary artery disease	+Ach with no epicardial narrowing but with reproduction of anginal chest pain but without ECG changes	Yes	Clopidogrel and ASA for 1 mo, ASA thereafter	No symptoms at 6 mo follow-up

4	51F (sister of case 1 and 2) with migraine and history of 2v CABG for SCAD, with recurrent angina	Yes	Yes, after CABG for presumed SCAD (initial diagnosis made at OSH)	TCD with 4/5 right-to-left shunt	Mild luminal irregularities in the epicardial coronary arteries with atretic left internal mammary artery- left anterior descending artery and absent radial-left circumflex artery	+Ach with narrowing of LAD	Yes	Clopidogrel and ASA for 1 mo, none since	No symptoms at 13 y follow-up; closed 2010
5	50F with migraines with visual aura, TND (right arm numbness and weakness, with right paralysis) and several months of angina	Yes, with visual aura	Yes	TEE with right-to-left shunting	N/A	N/A	Yes	Metoprolol	• No angina at 4 y follow-up • Reduced visual auras (from 20–30 episodes/y to <6 episodes/y)
6	34F with mixed connective tissue disorder, recurrent migraines and several months of angina	Yes, with aura	Yes	• TCD with 5/5 left-to-right shunt • TEE with left-to-right shunting	No epicardial atherosclerosis, mild myocardial bridge in the distal LAD	+Ach with >90% narrowing	Deferred in favor of clopidogrel therapy, now pending PFO closure	Clopidogrel	• Angina (15 d/mo) despite clopidogrel use at 5 mo follow-up with skin bruising • Mild improvement in migraines with aura

(continued on next page)

Table 1
(continued)

	Case Presentation	Migraines	Chest Pain	PFO Evaluation	Angiography	Provocative Testing	PFO Closure	Medical Therapy	Residual Symptoms/ Length of Follow-up
7	43F with migraines with visual aura, TND symptoms, factor V Leiden, and recurrent episodes of angina (3–5 × per week, improved with nitroglycerin)	Yes, with visual aura	Yes, nitrate responsive	TEE with right-to-left shunt and atrial septal aneurysm	N/A	N/A	Pending	Clopidogrel Nitroglycerin spray PRN	• Improvement in angina with nitroglycerin and clopidogrel with no improvement in migraine • Has transitioned to ticagrelor with improvement in migraine
8	47F with hypertension, obesity, IDDM, OSA, migraine, hypoxemia, and recurrent angina	Yes	Yes	• TEE with right-to-left shunt • Large shunt reported on TCD	No epicardial coronary artery disease	+Ach with narrowing of LAD	Yes	• Clopidogrel + ASA followed by ASA monotherapy • Currently on diltiazem, losartan, and rosuvastatin	• Occasional angina subsequently (2–3 × per month) • Improvement in migraine (now with 20/y) • 4 y follow-up, closed 2019
9	65F with supraventricular tachycardia, asthma, and HCV with several years of angina	No	Yes	TTE bubble study with right-to-left shunt	No epicardial coronary artery disease	+Ach with narrowing of diagonal artery	Surgical closure	ASA, Imdur, SL nitroglycerin PRN	• Minimal angina with antianginal therapy • Reports significant improvement in functional capacity • 4 y follow-up, closed 2019

the vasoactive substances may be cleared. Further systematic investigations with randomized controlled trials are warranted.

TAKOTSUBO SYNDROME AND CORONARY VASOSPASM

Coronary vasospasm has also been implicated in the pathogenesis of Takotsubo cardiomyopathy. Proposed mechanisms for the development of Takotsubo cardiomyopathy include spasm in response to increased autonomic tone or other stimulus resulting in increased levels of catecholamines, microvascular spasm, and neuroendocrine stimulation resulting in myocardial toxicity.[27,28] That Takotsubo is associated with elevated serum catecholamine and stress neuropeptide levels is well established. However, recent studies have implicated endothelial dysfunction resulting in coronary vasospasm as another underlying process contributing to Takotsubo. Indeed, up to 21% of patients with Takotsubo develop coronary vasospasm with provocative testing.[27,29,30]

In a case series of 4 patients, Angelini and colleagues demonstrated severe narrowing of the coronary arteries in patients with left ventricular apical ballooning with provocation testing with acetylcholine.[31] One patient was noted to have reproduction of left ventricular apical ballooning during acetylcholine administration. Similarly, in a study of 30 patients with Takotsubo, Kurisu found that provocative testing resulted in simultaneous, multivessel coronary spasm in either the epicardial or microvascular vessels.[29] These findings strongly support vasospasm as a central process in the pathophysiology of Takotsubo cardiomyopathy.

Lastly, the fact that postmenopausal women are predisposed to Takotsubo cardiomyopathy may suggest estrogen-related endothelial dysfunction.[28] Animal studies have demonstrated the benefit of estrogen supplementation, in addition to alpha-adrenoreceptor and beta-adrenoreceptor blockers, in preventing Takotsubo.[28,32]

Considering that endothelial dysfunction and vasospasm are key factors in the development of Takotsubo cardiomyopathy, the presence of PFO may be an underlying pathway in the pathogenesis of Takotsubo cardiomyopathy. While this hypothesis has not been fully investigated, there have been case reports suggesting a link between PFO and Takotsubo cardiomyopathy. Takafuji reported a case of a 16-year-old patient with PFO who suffered embolic stroke and was found to have reverse Takotsubo cardiomyopathy, suggesting hyperreactivity of the coronary circulation resulting in Takotsubo cardiomyopathy.[33] Further investigation is warranted to elucidate the mechanistic relationship between PFO and Takotsubo syndrome. Evaluation for the presence of PFO may identify individuals at risk for the development of Takotsubo cardiomyopathy and patients who may benefit from prophylactic PFO closure.

In summary, PFO may play a significant role in the development of migraine, vasospastic angina, and Takotsubo cardiomyopathy. The diagnosis and management of chest pain contributes greatly to the cost of health care and leads to significant morbidity. While further research is necessary to fully elucidate the mechanistic link between PFO and these clinical symptoms, percutaneous closure of PFO has been demonstrated to reduce the burden of symptoms and improve quality of life. Further characterizing the clinical syndrome of PFO, vasospastic angina, and migraine, as well as the risk factors that predispose specific individuals to these symptoms may help identify individuals who would benefit from PFO closure. Moreover, early closure of PFO in susceptible individuals may prevent more severe sequelae, such as Takotsubo cardiomyopathy or paradoxical embolism.

CLINICS CARE POINTS

- Consider evaluating for PFO in patients with cryptogenic stroke and elevated rsk of paradoxical embolism (ROPE) score.
- Consider invasive coronary functional testing with acetylcholine in patients with angina and no evidence of obstructive coronary artery disease.
- Use results of invasive coronary functional testing to guide the medical management of ANOCA based on specific phenotype/likely underlying mechanism contributing to symptoms.
- In patients with ANOCA, obtain a transcranial Doppler study to determine if there is a right-to-left shunt through a PFO.

REFERENCES

1. Charles A. The pathophysiology of migraine: implications for clinical management. Lancet Neurol 2018;17(2):174–82.
2. Finocchi C, Del Sette M. Migraine with aura and patent foramen ovale: myth or reality? Neurol Sci 2015;36(1):61–6.

3. Ning M, Navaratna D, Demirjian Z, et al. How the heart whispers to the brain: serotonin as neurovascular mediator in patent foramen ovale related stroke. Stroke 2011;42(3):e108.

4. Tietjen GE, Collins SA. Hypercoagulability and migraine. Headache. The Journal of Head and Face Pain 2018;58(1):173–83.

5. Liu K, Wang BZ, Hao Y, et al. The correlation between migraine and patent foramen ovale. Front Neurol 2020;11:543485.

6. Lip ZYP, Lip YHG. Patent foramen ovale and migraine attacks: a systematic review. Am J Med 2014;127:411–20.

7. Schwedt TJ, Demaerschalk BM, Dodick DW. Patent foramen ovale and migraine: a quantitative systemic review. Cephalalgia 2008;28:531–40.

8. Schwerzmann M, Nedeltchev K, Lagger F, et al. Prevalence and size of directly detected patent foramen ovale in migraine with aura. Neurology 2005;65: 1415–8.

9. Anzola GP, Morandi E, Casilli F, et al. Different degrees of right-to-left shunting predict migraine and stroke: data from 420 patients. Neurology 2006;66: 765–7.

10. Guo Y, Shi Y, Zhu D, et al. Clopidogrel can be an effective complementary prophylactic for drug-refractory migraine with patent foramen ovale. J Investig Med 2020;68(7):1250–5.

11. Wang F, Cao Y, Liu Y, et al. Platelet p2y12 inhibitor in the treatment and prevention of migraine: a systematic review and meta-analysis. Behav Neurol 2022; 2022:2118740.

12. Rodés-Cabau J, Horlick E, Ibrahim R, et al. Effect of clopidogrel and aspirin vs aspirin alone on migraine headaches after transcatheter atrial septal defect closure: the canoa randomized clinical trial. JAMA 2015;314(20):2147–54.

13. Dowson A, Mullen MJ, Peatfield R, et al. Migraine intervention with starflex technology (Mist) trial: a prospective, multicenter, double-blind, sham-controlled trial to evaluate the effectiveness of patent foramen ovale closure with starflex septal repair implant to resolve refractory migraine headache. Circulation 2008;117(11): 1397–404.

14. Mattle HP, Evers S, Hildick-Smith D, et al. Percutaneous closure of patent foramen ovale in migraine with aura, a randomized controlled trial. Eur Heart J 2016;37(26):2029–36.

15. Tobis J, Charles A, Silberstein S, et al. Percutaneous closure of patent foramen ovale in patients with migraine: the PREMIUM trial. J Am Coll Cardiol 2017;70(22):2766–74.

16. Mojadidi M, Kumar P, Mahmoud A, et al. Pooled analysis of PFO occluder device trials in patients with PFO and migraine. J Am Coll Cardiol 2021; 77(6):667–76.

17. Pepine C, Ferdinand K, Shaw L, et al. Emergence of Nonobstructive coronary artery disease: a Woman's Problem and need for change in Definition on angiography. J Am Coll Cardiol 2015;66(17): 1918–33.

18. Ford Thomas J, Stanley Bethany, Richard Good, et al. Stratified medical therapy using invasive coronary function testing in angina. J Am Coll Cardiol 2018;72(23_Part_A):2841–55.

19. Kent DM, Ruthazer R, Weimar C, et al. An index to identify stroke-related vs incidental patent foramen ovale in cryptogenic stroke. Neurology 2013;81(7): 619–25.

20. Matta A, Bouisset F, Lhermusier T, et al. Coronary artery spasm: new insights. J Interv Cardiol 2020; 2020:5894586.

21. Jansen T, Konst R, Elias-Smale S, et al. Assessing microvascular dysfunction in angina with Unobstructed coronary arteries: JACC review Topic of the Week. J Am Coll Cardiol 2021;78(14):1471–9.

22. Minoca from a to z. American College of Cardiology.2022. Available at: https://www.acc.org/Latest-in-Cardiology/Articles/2022/01/05/17/41/MINOCA-from-A-to-Z.

23. Pries AR, Badimon L, Bugiardini R, et al. Coronary vascular regulation, remodelling, and collateralization: mechanisms and clinical implications on behalf of the working group on coronary pathophysiology and microcirculation. Eur Heart J 2015;36(45): 3134–46.

24. Feenstra R, Seitz A, Boerhout C, et al. Principles and pitfalls in coronary vasomotor function testing. EuroIntervention 2022;17(15):1271–80.

25. Knuuti J, Wijns W, Saraste A, et al. 2019 ESC Guidelines for the diagnosis and management of chronic coronary syndromes. Eur Heart J 2020;41(3): 407–77.

26. Ravi D, Parikh R, Aboulhosn J, et al. A new syndrome of patent foramen ovale inducing vasospastic angina and migraine. JACC (J Am Coll Cardiol): Case Reports 2023;28:102132.

27. Tsuchihashi K, Ueshima K, Uchida T, et al. Transient left ventricular apical ballooning without coronary artery stenosis: a novel heart syndrome mimicking acute myocardial infarction. J Am Coll Cardiol 2001;38(1):11–8.

28. Pelliccia F, Kaski JC, Crea F, et al. Pathophysiology of takotsubo syndrome. Circulation 2017;135(24): 2426–41.

29. Kurisu S, Sato H, Kawagoe T, et al. Tako-tsubo-like left ventricular dysfunction with ST-segment elevation: a novel cardiac syndrome mimicking acute myocardial infarction. Am Heart J 2002;143(3): 448–55.

30. Angelini P, Uribe C, Tobis JM. Pathophysiology of takotsubo cardiomyopathy: reopened debate. Tex Heart Inst J 2021;48(3):e207490.

31. Angelini P. Transient left ventricular apical ballooning: a unifying pathophysiologic theory at the edge of Prinzmetal angina. Cathet Cardiovasc Intervent 2008;71(3):342–52.

32. Ueyama T, Ishikura F, Matsuda A, et al. Chronic estrogen supplementation following ovariectomy improves the emotional stress-induced cardiovascular responses by indirect action on the nervous system and by direct action on the heart. Circ J 2007;71(4): 565–73.

33. Takafuji H, Arai J, Saigusa K, et al. Reverse takotsubo cardiomyopathy caused by patent foramen ovale-related cryptogenic stroke: a case report. Eur Heart J Case Rep 2020;4(6):1–6.

UNITED STATES POSTAL SERVICE®

Statement of Ownership, Management, and Circulation
(All Periodicals Publications Except Requester Publications)

1. Publication Title	2. Publication Number	3. Filing Date
CARDIOLOGY CLINICS	000 – 701	9/18/2024

4. Issue Frequency	5. Number of Issues Published Annually	6. Annual Subscription Price
FEB, MAY, AUG, NOV	4	$396.00

7. Complete Mailing Address of Known Office of Publication (Not printer) (Street, city, county, state, and ZIP+4®)

ELSEVIER INC.
230 Park Avenue, Suite 800
New York, NY 10169

Contact Person: Malathi Samayan
Telephone (Include area code): 91-44-4299-4507

8. Complete Mailing Address of Headquarters or General Business Office of Publisher (Not printer)

ELSEVIER INC.
230 Park Avenue, Suite 800
New York, NY 10169

9. Full Names and Complete Mailing Addresses of Publisher, Editor, and Managing Editor (Do not leave blank)

Publisher (Name and complete mailing address)
Dolores Meloni, ELSEVIER INC.
1600 JOHN F KENNEDY BLVD. SUITE 1600
PHILADELPHIA, PA 19103-2899

Editor (Name and complete mailing address)
JOANNA GASCOINE, ELSEVIER INC.
1600 JOHN F KENNEDY BLVD. SUITE 1600
PHILADELPHIA, PA 19103-2899

Managing Editor (Name and complete mailing address)
PATRICK MANLEY, ELSEVIER INC.
1600 JOHN F KENNEDY BLVD. SUITE 1600
PHILADELPHIA, PA 19103-2899

10. Owner (Do not leave blank. If the publication is owned by a corporation, give the name and address of the corporation immediately followed by the names and addresses of all stockholders owning or holding 1 percent or more of the total amount of stock. If not owned by a corporation, give the names and addresses of the individual owners. If owned by a partnership or other unincorporated firm, give its name and address as well as those of each individual owner. If the publication is published by a nonprofit organization, give its name and address.)

Full Name	Complete Mailing Address
WHOLLY OWNED SUBSIDIARY OF REED/ELSEVIER, US HOLDINGS	1600 JOHN F KENNEDY BLVD. SUITE 1600 PHILADELPHIA, PA 19103-2899

11. Known Bondholders, Mortgagees, and Other Security Holders Owning or Holding 1 Percent or More of Total Amount of Bonds, Mortgages, or Other Securities. If none, check box ▶ ☐ None

Full Name	Complete Mailing Address
N/A	

12. Tax Status (For completion by nonprofit organizations authorized to mail at nonprofit rates) (Check one)
The purpose, function, and nonprofit status of this organization and the exempt status for federal income tax purposes:
☒ Has Not Changed During Preceding 12 Months
☐ Has Changed During Preceding 12 Months (Publisher must submit explanation of change with this statement)

PS Form **3526**, July 2014 (Page 1 of 4 (see instructions page 4)) PSN: 7530-01-000-9931 PRIVACY NOTICE: See our privacy policy on www.usps.com.

13. Publication Title	14. Issue Date for Circulation Data Below
CARDIOLOGY CLINICS	AUGUST 2024

15. Extent and Nature of Circulation			Average No. Copies Each Issue During Preceding 12 Months	No. Copies of Single Issue Published Nearest to Filing Date
a. Total Number of Copies (Net press run)			133	138
b. Paid Circulation (By Mail and Outside the Mail)	(1)	Mailed Outside-County Paid Subscriptions Stated on PS Form 3541 (Include paid distribution above nominal rate, advertiser's proof copies, and exchange copies)	79	82
	(2)	Mailed In-County Paid Subscriptions Stated on PS Form 3541 (Include paid distribution above nominal rate, advertiser's proof copies, and exchange copies)	0	0
	(3)	Paid Distribution Outside the Mails Including Sales Through Dealers and Carriers, Street Vendors, Counter Sales, and Other Paid Distribution Outside USPS®	41	42
	(4)	Paid Distribution by Other Classes of Mail Through the USPS (e.g., First-Class Mail®)	5	5
c. Total Paid Distribution (Sum of 15b (1), (2), (3), and (4))			125	129
d. Free or Nominal Rate Distribution (By Mail and Outside the Mail)	(1)	Free or Nominal Rate Outside-County Copies included on PS Form 3541	7	8
	(2)	Free or Nominal Rate In-County Copies Included on PS Form 3541	0	0
	(3)	Free or Nominal Rate Copies Mailed at Other Classes Through the USPS (e.g., First-Class Mail)	0	0
	(4)	Free or Nominal Rate Distribution Outside the Mail (Carriers or other means)	1	1
e. Total Free or Nominal Rate Distribution (Sum of 15d (1), (2), (3) and (4))			8	9
f. Total Distribution (Sum of 15c and 15e)			133	138
g. Copies not Distributed (See Instructions to Publishers #4 (page #3))			0	0
h. Total (Sum of 15f and g)			133	138
i. Percent Paid (15c divided by 15f times 100)			94.16%	93.48%

* If you are claiming electronic copies, go to line 16 on page 3. If you are not claiming electronic copies, skip to line 17 on page 3.

PS Form **3526**, July 2014 (Page 2 of 4)

16. Electronic Copy Circulation	Average No. Copies Each Issue During Preceding 12 Months	No. Copies of Single Issue Published Nearest to Filing Date
a. Paid Electronic Copies ▶		
b. Total Paid Print Copies (Line 15c) + Paid Electronic Copies (Line 16a) ▶		
c. Total Print Distribution (Line 15f) + Paid Electronic Copies (Line 16a) ▶		
d. Percent Paid (Both Print & Electronic Copies) (16b divided by 16c × 100) ▶		

☒ I certify that 50% of all my distributed copies (electronic and print) are paid above a nominal price.

17. Publication of Statement of Ownership

☒ If the publication is a general publication, publication of this statement is required. Will be printed in the NOVEMBER 2024 issue of this publication. ☐ Publication not required.

18. Signature and Title of Editor, Publisher, Business Manager, or Owner

Malathi Samayan

Malathi Samayan - Distribution Controller

Date: 9/18/2024

I certify that all information furnished on this form is true and complete. I understand that anyone who furnishes false or misleading information on this form or who omits material or information requested on the form may be subject to criminal sanctions (including fines and imprisonment) and/or civil sanctions (including civil penalties).

PS Form **3526**, July 2014 (Page 3 of 4) PRIVACY NOTICE: See our privacy policy on www.usps.com.

Moving?

Make sure your subscription moves with you!

To notify us of your new address, find your **Clinics Account Number** (located on your mailing label above your name), and contact customer service at:

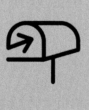

Email: journalscustomerservice-usa@elsevier.com

800-654-2452 (subscribers in the U.S. & Canada)
314-447-8871 (subscribers outside of the U.S. & Canada)

Fax number: 314-447-8029

Elsevier Health Sciences Division
Subscription Customer Service
3251 Riverport Lane
Maryland Heights, MO 63043

*To ensure uninterrupted delivery of your subscription, please notify us at least 4 weeks in advance of move.

Printed and bound by CPI Group (UK) Ltd, Croydon, CR0 4YY

08/05/2025

01864747-0009